Life Care Planning

Editors

MICHEL LACERTE
CLOIE B. JOHNSON

PHYSICAL MEDICINE AND REHABILITATION CLINICS OF NORTH AMERICA

www.pmr.theclinics.com

Consulting Editor
GREGORY T. CARTER

August 2013 • Volume 24 • Number 3

ELSEVIER

1600 John F. Kennedy Boulevard • Suite 1800 • Philadelphia, Pennsylvania, 19103-2899

http://www.theclinics.com

PHYSICAL MEDICINE AND REHABILITATION CLINICS OF NORTH AMERICA Volume 24, Number 3
August 2013 ISSN 1047-9651, ISBN-978-0-323-18615-5

Editor: Jessica McCool

Reprints. For copies of 100 or more of articles in this publication, please contact the Commercial Reprints
Department, Elsevier Inc., 360 Park Avenue South, New York, NY 10010-1710. Tel.: 212-633-3812; Fax:
212-462-1935; E-mail: reprints@elsevier.com.

Physical Medicine and Rehabilitation Clinics of North America (ISSN 1047-9651) is published quarterly by
Elsevier Inc., 360 Park Avenue South, New York, NY 10010-1710. Months of issue are February, May,
August, and November. Business and Editorial Offices: 1600 John F. Kennedy Blvd., Suite 1800, Philadelphia,
PA 19103-2899. Customer Service Office: 3251 Riverport Lane, Maryland Heights, MO 63043. Periodicals post-
age paid at New York, NY and additional mailing offices. Subscription price per year is $263.00 (US individuals),
$459.00 (US institutions), $140.00 (US students), $320.00 (Canadian individuals), $598.00 (Canadian institu-
tions), $200.00 (Canadian students), $395.00 (foreign individuals), $598.00 (foreign institutions), and $200.00
(foreign students). Foreign air speed delivery is included in all *Clinics* subscription prices. All prices are subject
to change without notice. POSTMASTER: Send address changes to *Physical Medicine and Rehabilitation
Clinics of North America*, Customer Service Office: Elsevier Health Sciences Division, Subscription Customer
Service, 3251 Riverport Lane, Maryland Heights, MO 63043. **Customer Service: 1-800-654-2452 (US).
From outside of the United States, call 314-447-8871. Fax: 314-447-8029. E-mail: JournalsCustomer
Service-usa@elsevier.com (for print support); JournalsOnlineSupport-usa@elsevier.com (for online
support).**

Physical Medicine and Rehabilitation Clinics of North America is indexed in *Excerpta Medica, MEDLINE/
PubMed (Index Medicus), Cinahl,* and *Cumulative Index to Nursing and Allied Health Literature.*

Printed and bound by CPI Group (UK) Ltd, Croydon, CR0 4YY
Transferred to digital print 2013

Contributors

CONSULTING EDITOR

GREGORY T. CARTER, MD, MS
Medical Director, Muscular Dystrophy Association Regional Neuromuscular Center, Providence Medical Group, Department of Clinical Neurosciences; Physical Medicine and Rehabilitation Division, Olympia, Washington

EDITORS

MICHEL LACERTE, MDCM, MSc, FRCPC, CCRC
Co-Chair, Canadian Life Care Planning Summit 2011; Founding Member, Canadian Society of Medical Evaluators; Associate Professor, Department of Physical Medicine and Rehabilitation, Schulich School of Medicine and Dentistry, Western University, London, Ontario; Associate Director, Insurance Medicine and Medico-legal Expertise Diploma Program, Université de Montréal, Montreal, Quebec, Canada

CLOIE B. JOHNSON, MEd, ABVE-D, CCM
Co-Chair, Life Care Planning Summit 2010, Co-Chair, Canadian Life Care Planning Summit 2011, Chair, Life Care Planning Summit 2012, Rehabilitation Counselor/Case Manager, OSC Vocational Systems, Inc, Bothell, Washington; Past Chair, International Academy of Life Care Planners/International Association of Rehabilitation Professionals, Glenview, Illinois

AUTHORS

ARTHUR AMEIS, BSC, MD, FRCPC, DESS, FAAPM&R (SUBSPECIALTY CERT PAIN MEDICINE)
Senior Medical Consultant, Arthur Ameis Medicine Professional Corporation, Toronto, Ontario; Lecturer, Certification Program in Insurance Medicine and MedicoLegal Expertise, Faculty of Medicine, Universite de Montreal, Montreal, Quebec, Canada

GREGORY T. CARTER, MD, MS
Medical Director, Muscular Dystrophy Association Regional Neuromuscular Center, Providence Medical Group, Department of Clinical Neurosciences; Physical Medicine and Rehabilitation Division, Olympia, Washington

ANTHONY J. CHOPPA, MEd, CRC, CCM, CDMS
Founder, OSC Vocational Systems, Inc, Bothell, Washington; Past International Academy of Life Care Planners Board Representative, International Association of Rehabilitation Professionals, Glenview, Illinois

HEIDI L. FAWBER, MEd, LPC, CRC, CCM, CLCP
Rehabilitation Consultant, Mars, Pennsylvania; International Association of Rehabilitation Professionals; International Academy of Life Care Planners Section, Glenview, Illinois

REG L. GIBBS, MS, CRC, LCPC, CBIS, CLCP
Founder, Rocky Mountain Rehab, P.C. and Brightsun Technologies Inc; Part-Time Instructor, Montana State University, Billings, Montana

FRANK K. JACKSON IV, MS
Arizona College of Osteopathic Medicine, Midwestern University, Glendale, Arizona

SIMONE P. JAVAHER, RN, BSN, MPA
Director, Division of Pain Medicine, Department of Anesthesiology and Pain Medicine, University of Washington School of Medicine, Seattle, Washington

CLOIE B. JOHNSON, MEd, ABVE-D, CCM
Co-Chair, Life Care Planning Summit 2010, Co-Chair, Canadian Life Care Planning Summit 2011, Chair, Life Care Planning Summit 2012, Rehabilitation Counselor/Case Manager, OSC Vocational Systems, Inc, Bothell, Washington; Past Chair, International Academy of Life Care Planners/International Association of Rehabilitation Professionals, Glenview, Illinois

RICHARD T. KATZ, MD
Professor of Clinical Neurology (Physical Medicine and Rehabilitation), Washington University School of Medicine, St Louis, Missouri

MICHEL LACERTE, MDCM, MSc, FRCPC, CCRC
Co-Chair, Canadian Life Care Planning Summit 2011; Founding Member, Canadian Society of Medical Evaluators, Toronto; Associate Professor, Department of Physical Medicine and Rehabilitation, Schulich School of Medicine and Dentistry, Western University, London, Ontario; Associate Director, Insurance Medicine and Medico-legal Expertise Diploma Program, Université de Montréal, Montreal, Quebec, Canada

ROBERT H. MEIER III, MD
Director, Amputee Services of America, Denver, Colorado; Fellow, American Academy of Physical Medicine and Rehabilitation, Rosemont, Illinois; Adjunct Faculty, St. Petersburg College, College of Orthotics and Prosthetics, St. Petersburg, Florida

SONIA PAQUETTE, OTD, OTR/L, CPE, ABVE-D
Private Litigation Consultant, Ergonomics and Vocational Rehabilitation, Downingtown, Pennsylvania; Physical Therapy Doctorate Program; Occupational Therapy Transitional Doctorate Program, Assistant Professor, Rocky Mountain University of Health Professions, Provo, Utah; Adjunct Faculty, Master's and Doctorate Programs, Occupational Therapy, Salus University, Elkins Park, Pennsylvania

JUDITH P. PARKER, MEd, CDMS, ABVE-D, CLCP
OSC Vocational Systems, Inc, Bothell, Washington

SUSAN N. RIDDICK-GRISHAM, RN, BA, CCM, CLCP
Founder, The Care Planner Network; Founder, Life Care Manager, Richmond, Virginia; Vice-Chair, Foundation for Life Care Planning Research, Oviedo, Florida; Advisory Board, Sarah Jane Brain Project, New York, New York; Board of Directors, International Association of Rehabilitation Professionals, Glenview, Illinois

RICK ROBINSON, PhD, MBA, LMHC, CRC, CVE, CLCP, D/ABVE, NCC
President, Robinson Work Rehabilitation Services Co, Jacksonville; Faculty Lecturer, Department of Behavioral Science and Community Health, University of Florida, Gainesville, Florida

BILL S. ROSEN, MD
Montana Neuroscience Institute, Montana Brain Injury Center, St. Patrick Hospital, Missoula, Montana

FRANÇOIS SESTIER, MD, PhD
Program Director, Faculty of Medicine, Insurance Medicine and Medicolegal Expertise, Université de Montréal, Montréal, Québec, Canada

STEVEN A. STIENS, MD, MS
Associate Professor, Department Rehabilitation Medicine; Fellowship Director, Spinal Cord Medicine, 2001-2012, University of Washington; Attending Physician, Spinal Cord Injury Unit, VA Puget Sound Health Care System, University Hospital; Board Member, Model Systems in Spinal Cord Injury, University of Washington, Seattle, Washington

PIERRE J. VACHON, PhD, JD, MPH
Principal, Life Expectancy Consulting, Sunnyvale, California

ROGER O. WEED, PhD
Professor Emeritus, Georgia State University, Atlanta, Georgia; Board Member Emeritus, Foundation for Life Care Planning Research; Past President, International Association of Rehabilitation Professionals, Glenview, Illinois

STEVEN A. YUHAS, MEd, CRC, CLCP, CCM, NCC, CBIS
Rehabilitation Consultant, Founder and President, The Directions Group, Inc, Mount Pleasant, South Carolina; International Academy of Life Care Planners Section; International Association of Rehabilitation Professionals, Glenview, Illinois

NATHAN D. ZASLER, MD
CEO and Medical Director, Concussion Care Centre of Virginia, Ltd; CEO and Medical Director, Tree of Life Services, Inc, Richmond, Virginia

Contents

This article discusses the history and evolution of what is now known as a life care plan. The qualifications of professionals who perform the specialty practice of life care planning are reviewed. The standards of practice for life care planning have been a long-standing guide for the practitioner and its core components are discussed.

The sequela of spinal cord injury (SCI) can provide a prototype for life care planning because the segmental design of the vertebrate body allows assessments to be quantitative, repeatable, and predictive of the injured person's impairments, self-care capabilities, and required assistance. Life care planning for patients with SCI uses a standard method that is comparable between planner, yet individualizes assessment and seeks resources that meet unique patient-centered needs in their communities of choice. Clinical care and rehabilitation needs organized with an SCI problem list promotes collaboration by the interdisciplinary team, caregivers, and family in efficient achievement of patient-centered goals and completion of daily care plans.

A life care plan is a detailed and comprehensive analysis of impairments, realistic needs, and associated costs relevant to providing a lifetime of care to patients. Physicians have a central role in advising life care planners. Within an expertly prepared life care plan, issues must correspond directly with proposed goods and services. A life care plan must clearly cite all relevant caregiver sources and rely on scientific evidence. The central tenets of a life care plan and the ethical and professional roles that physicians may play in the context of traumatic brain injury and a life care plan are reviewed in this article.

> Expert opinion on life expectancy must make reasonable factual assumptions, which entails finding a proper group to which the individual being assessed will be compared, as well as use of appropriate and reliable technical methods. Reasonable judgment should be exercised in the selection of the studies employed. A schedule of mortality rates must be built on a fair assessment of the person's medical condition and of relevant peer-reviewed findings. A clear and detailed report should be produced, containing the basis for the opinion, the description of the methods employed, and the life-expectancy calculations specific to the individual.

> This article outlines the use of medical literature to support a physiatrist's expert opinion in the development of a life care plan and proposes a basic ethical code of conduct in performing medicolegal work.

Life Care Planning

PHYSICAL MEDICINE & REHABILITATION CLINICS OF NORTH AMERICA

Foreword

Life Care Planning

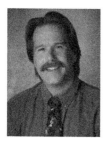

Gregory T. Carter, MD, MS
Consulting Editor

After suffering a life-altering, typically life-threatening event, a patient is left facing an uncertain, unclear future, entering a new, previously unforeseen, world. Following a catastrophic injury, perhaps a brain or spinal cord injury, there is typically an initial period of crisis where a patient may be clinging to life in an intensive care unit (ICU), kept alive with the assistance of ventilators and intravenous medications and nutrition. From there, the patient begins the road to rehabilitation, often done still in the hospital setting in an in-patient unit. Here is often where other injuries now become more apparent, including bone and joint injuries that may have been wholly missed previously. The patient's day begins with the smiling face of a physical therapist, and new aches and pains. Still the day is planned and the calendar is full, with a minimum of options. The therapeutic choices are limited at this point and the goal is mainly to go home. This is the point where the patient may recall first meeting the physiatrist, although often we do see the patient even in the ICU.

Finally the day comes when the patient is discharged from the in-patient setting, back "home"…yet home is now a very different place. Home may not have changed much, yet the patient has, perhaps now needing a wheelchair for mobility. What lies ahead? What do the next 20, 30, or even 40 years hold in store? Enter Life Care Planning.

Thanks to the dedicated efforts of my friend and physiatry colleague, Michel Lacerte, MD, and his co-guest editor, Cloie B. Johnson, MEd, ABVE, CCM, we have before us a remarkably well-done issue of the *Physical Medicine and Rehabilitation Clinics of North America* devoted entirely to Life Care Planning. This issue focuses

Phys Med Rehabil Clin N Am 24 (2013) xi–xiii
http://dx.doi.org/10.1016/j.pmr.2013.03.011
1047-9651/13/$ – see front matter © 2013 Published by Elsevier Inc.

pmr.theclinics.com

exactly on the "What lies ahead?" part, including the long-term comprehensive care of a patient suffering from the consequences of a major catastrophic life event, including limb loss, traumatic spinal cord and brain injury, cerebral palsy, and spinal and neuropathic pain. Also covered herein is an overview of the life care planning process with particular attention to the role of the physiatrist in this process, as well as discussions on life expectancy determination, work life expectancy, and vocational rehabilitation.

Michel and Cloie bring a wealth of experience to this project and have recruited some of the top names in this field to fill out the roster. This includes several people whom I am honored to count as very close personal friends. Dr Robert "Skip" Meier III has been a friend and mentor for me throughout my entire career, going back to residency training. This brings up Dr Bill S. Rosen, who is another dear friend. Bill and I were residents together. We were both fortunate to have benefited from Dr Meier's teaching because he would fly in from Denver to teach prosthetics and care of the amputee to our residency classmates. Dr Meier covers life care planning for the amputee, joined by certified Life Care Planner, Anthony J. Choppa, and our guest editor Cloie B. Johnson, MEd, ABVE, CCM. Dr Rosen is joined by life care planner Reg L. Gibbs and Dr Lacerte to give us an excellent overview of the published research in this field, a very useful article.

The issue starts out with a nice introduction to the life care planning process by editor, Cloie B. Johnson, and Roger O. Weed, a professor of vocational rehabilitation at Georgia State University, and an enormously well-published academician. Joining this esteemed group is another good buddy from Seattle, Dr Steve Steins, a renowned expert in spinal cord medicine, and his coauthors, Heidi L. Fawber, MEd, CRC, CCM, CLCP, and Steven A. Yuhas. They cover all aspects of life care planning for patients with spinal cord injury.

Life care planning for children with cerebral palsy is thoroughly addressed by senior physiatrist and bona fide expert Dr Richard T. Katz, joined by our editor, Cloie B. Johnson. I was very honored to join my dear friends, Simone P. Javaher, RN, BSN, MPA, Frank K. Jackson, BS, MS IV, and Judith P. Parker, Med, to cover the many aspects of neuropathic pain, which must be considered in doing life care planning. Simone and I have worked on many projects together, and, as always, she was invaluable to the success of our article. Frank Jackson has been a mentee of mine for years and is currently finishing medical school and will be pursuing physiatry training at the University of Utah. Judith Parker, a certified life care planner, was the glue that held us together! Rounding out our issue is an excellent treatise on the vocational rehabilitation process as it pertains to work life by Dr Rick Robinson, a nationally recognized rehabilitation counselor, vocational evaluator, and life care planner, and Dr Sonia Paquette, a work and functional capacity expert who has expertise in vocational potential, loss of earnings capacity, and transferable skills analysis. The issue closes with another excellent article on determining life expectancy by Pierre J. Vachon, PhD, MPH, an expert in epidemiology and population demographics joined by Dr François Sestier, a Clinical Professor of Medicine, University of Montreal, Faculty of Medicine, and an expert in human morbidity and mortality. I am personally very grateful to all of the authors who contributed hours of dedicated work here. I also want to express my personal gratitude to our editors, Michel Lacerte and Cloie B. Johnson, for going the extra mile to make this a high-quality finished product. Finally I offer a special thanks to our always patient editor, Jessica McCool, from Elsevier.

I would like to personally dedicate this book to the countless numbers of catastrophically injured patients we have all cared for over the years. These patients continue to amaze us all, revealing the remarkable perseverance of the human spirit to push onward, even in the face of unspeakable misfortune and pain.

Gregory T. Carter, MD, MS
Muscular Dystrophy Association
Regional Neuromuscular Center
Providence Medical Group
Department of Clinical Neurosciences
Physical Medicine and Rehabilitation Division
410 Providence Lane, Building 2
Olympia, WA 98506, USA

E-mail address:
gtcarter@uw.edu

Preface

Life Care Planning

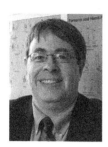 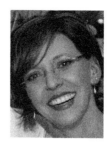

Michel Lacerte, MDCM, MSc, FRCPC, CCRC   Cloie B. Johnson, MEd, ABVE-D, CCM
Editors

Physiatrists have long been recognized as uniquely qualified among medical specialists to provide the scientific and medical foundation essential to the development of life care plans. Physiatrists experienced in the medical management of individuals with catastrophic injuries are often relied on by life care planners to establish future care needs along with expected complications, including functional deterioration, while taking into account the particular context of the individual with a disability.

While most physiatrists are aware of life care planning and life expectancy determination concepts in personal injury litigation, few have been adequately trained in the foundation process and nuances in litigation to face deposition and courtroom challenges. Working in a close relationship with experienced life care planners will facilitate the presentation of reasonable needs and associated costs according to life care planning standards of practice.

This *Physical Medicine and Rehabilitation Clinics of North America* issue is the result of a close collaboration of physiatrists and life care planners; such collaboration is necessary to successfully manage patients with catastrophic impairments or complex health care needs. Evidence-based medicine and comparative effectiveness research must also be part of the mix for life care plans to meet the scientific evidence admissibility standards in courts.

This work would have not been possible without the exceptional technical editorial support from Mr Joseph Petrik. We wish to thank Dr Greg Carter and Mrs Jessica McCool from Elsevier for giving this outstanding group of authors the opportunity to work together on this project. We hope it will generate interest in the field and

Phys Med Rehabil Clin N Am 24 (2013) xv–xvi
http://dx.doi.org/10.1016/j.pmr.2013.03.010
1047-9651/13/$ – see front matter © 2013 Published by Elsevier Inc.

pmr.theclinics.com

encourage our readers to consider life care planning as an important field for future physical medicine and rehabilitation research and collaboration.

Michel Lacerte, MDCM, MSc, FRCPC, CCRC
Department of Physical Medicine and Rehabilitation
Schulich School of Medicine & Dentistry
Western University
London, Ontario, Canada

4520 Colonel Talbot Road, Box 10
Lambeth Station
London, Ontario, Canada N6P 1P9

Cloie B. Johnson, MEd, ABVE-D, CCM
OSC Vocational Systems Inc
10132 NE 185th Street
Bothell, WA 98011, USA

International Academy of Life Care Planners/
International Association of Rehabilitation Professionals
1926 Waukegan Road, Suite 1
Glenview, IL 60025-1770, USA

E-mail addresses:
mlacerte@uwo.ca (M. Lacerte)
cloie@osc-voc.com (C.B. Johnson)

The Life Care Planning Process

Cloie B. Johnson, MEd, ABVE-D, CCM[a,b,c,]*, Roger O. Weed, PhD[c,d,e]

KEYWORDS

- Life care plan • Case management • Standards of practice • Qualifications

KEY POINTS

- A life care plan is a tool of case management.
- A life care plan is based on proper medical, psychological, case management, and rehabilitation foundation.
- The development of a life care plan requires following generally accepted and peer-reviewed methodology and standards of practice.
- Life care planning is a transdisciplinary specialty practice.
- A life care plan is a dynamic document based on published standards of practice, comprehensive assessment, data analysis, and research that provides an organized concise plan for current and future needs with associated costs for individuals who have experienced catastrophic injury or have chronic health care needs.

INTRODUCTION

A life care plan is a tool of case management, used for medical treatment planning and management purposes in many venues.[1] Understanding what a life care plan is, how it is created, and the various roles of the rehabilitation counselor, case manager, or other professional coordinating a life care plan along with his or her integral role in compiling a life care plan are the focus of this article. A life care plan is based on proper medical, psychological, case management, and rehabilitation foundation.[2,3] Life care plans require consistently applied methodology, combined with professional clinical judgment.[4]

Clinical judgment is the embodiment of a clinician's experiences, and throughout the process of coordinating and implementing a life care plan clinical judgment is used to ensure that the life care plan is specific and appropriate to the individual.[4]

Funding Sources: None.
Conflict of Interest: None.
[a] International Academy of Life Care Planners, 1926 Waukegan Road, Suite 1, Glenview, IL 60025-1770, USA; [b] OSC Vocational Systems Inc, 10132 Northeast 185th Street, Bothell, WA 98011; [c] International Association of Rehabilitation Professionals, 1926 Waukegan Road, Suite 1, Glenview, IL 60025-1770, USA; [d] Georgia State University, 30, Courtland Street SE, Atlanta, GA 30303, USA; [e] Foundation for Life Care Planning Research, 10 Windsormere Way Ste. 400 Oviedo, FL 3276, USA
* Corresponding author. OSC Vocational Systems Inc, 10132 Northeast 185th Street, Bothell, WA 98011.
E-mail address: cloie@osc-voc.com

Phys Med Rehabil Clin N Am 24 (2013) 403–417
http://dx.doi.org/10.1016/j.pmr.2013.03.008
1047-9651/13/$ – see front matter © 2013 Elsevier Inc. All rights reserved.

This article outlines the methodology, standards, and process to assist in educating readers if they are requested to provide a foundation for a life care plan.

HISTORY

Life care plans have evolved over time for multiple purposes.[5] Rehabilitation planning had its genesis in legislation beginning primarily in 1917 (Smith-Hughes Act), and it has continued to develop into the 1960s and 1970s as a result of major legislation that provided services for all people with disabilities.[6,7] In their seminal 1967 publication, McGowan and Porter[6] noted that the range of "modern day" rehabilitation services included full evaluation, counseling and guidance, medical services and care, prosthetics, vocational training, services through rehabilitation facilities, maintenance and transportation, tools and equipment, and placement services.

The major functions of the counselor require assuming responsibility to evaluate the client; planning with the individual from the initial counseling interview and diagnostic services to the establishment of eligibility, planning, and arranging the supervision of services; and being responsible for final job adjustment. Also included in these functions is responsibility for effective management of the caseload, case records, correspondence, reports, and workflow.[6]

Deutsch and Raffa[8] first established the guidelines to determine damages in civil litigation cases. By 1985, the *Guide to Rehabilitation* had introduced the life care plan to the health care industry.[2] Since 1985, when the life care plan first emerged in the rehabilitation literature, the concept has grown immensely and it is now the most effective case management method used within the industry, particularly with regard to complex and medically challenging cases.[9–13]

Life care plans have historically been used in a variety of settings, including managed care; workers' compensation claims; Medicare set-aside plans; in response to the Federal Employees Liability Act, Jones Act, Longshore and Harbor Workers' Compensation Act, and in Office of Workers Compensation Programs cases; and for dissolution litigation, personal injury litigation, employment litigation, mediation, reserve setting for insurance companies, federal vaccine injury fund cases, and family trusts.[14] Each venue has special life care planning considerations that are beyond the scope of this article.

The development of a comprehensive plan of care has always been an integral part of the medical and rehabilitation process. This type of plan has been used historically by multiple medically related disciplines. Rehabilitation professionals create a rehabilitation plan, nurses develop a nursing care plan,[15] physicians define a medical treatment plan,[3] and other professions develop plans specific to their practice.[14,16] Because of rapid growth in medical technology and an increased emphasis on the cost of care, including concepts of managed care, information on the specific cost of care has become an increasingly important aspect of health care. The process of developing a comprehensive plan and delineating costs has evolved over an extensive period and it is now used by case managers, counselors, and other professionals in many sectors. The life care plan represents an acceptable and pragmatic approach to the delivery of services within myriad sectors of the health care delivery system.

Rehabilitation or life care plans have been used in a variety of health care and legal settings to provide information and documentation on the cost of services related to long-term care.[17] These plans are also provided as valuable tools for such areas as rehabilitation planning; geriatric services implementation; and management of health care resources, discharge planning, educational planning, and long-term managed care.[18]

TRANSDISCIPLINARY PERSPECTIVE

Life care planning is a transdisciplinary specialty practice.[14,16] Each profession brings to the process of life care planning practice standards that must be adhered to by the individual professional, and these standards remain applicable while the practitioner engages in life care planning activities. Each professional works within specific standards and scope of practice for their discipline to ensure accountability, provide direction, and mandate responsibility for the standards for which they are accountable. These include, but are not limited to, activities related to quality of care, qualifications, collaboration, law, ethics, advocacy, resource use, and research.

In addition, individual practitioners must examine their qualifications as applied to each individual case. Therefore, thorough knowledge of the medical diagnosis, disability, and long-term care considerations, by virtue of education and experience, is a necessary component of the practitioner's competency for each case. Moreover, each practitioner is responsible for following the standards of practice for life care planning in addition to the standards for the practitioner's qualifying profession.

DEFINITION

A life care plan is a dynamic document based on published standards of practice, comprehensive assessment, data analysis, and research that provides an organized concise plan for current and future needs with associated costs for individuals who have experienced catastrophic injury or have chronic health care needs. This combined definition was derived from the University of Florida and Intellicus annual life care planning conference, and the American Academy of Nurse Life Care Planners (now known as the International Academy of Life Care Planners [IALCP]), presented at the Forensic Section meeting, National Association of Rehabilitation Professionals in the Private Sector annual conference, Colorado Springs, Colorado, and agreed on April 3, 1998, as cited in the IALCP Standards of Practice.[14,19]

The life care plan is developed in many instances to identify damages in civil cases involving liability.[8] However, the general content of the plan prepared by the coordinator and by the professional completing a life care plan are essentially the same: they detail what maintenance services and support items a person with a disability would need to achieve optimal recovery during the postinjury period.

The life care plan should be a working document that provides accurate and timely information that can be easily used by the client and interested parties. The plan should be updated as needed and serve as a lifelong guide to assist in the delivery of health care services in a managed format.

If possible, the life care plan should be a collaborative effort among the various parties and it should reflect preventive and rehabilitative goals. As a dynamic document, the life care plan requires periodic updating to accommodate changes and should have as its goal quality outcomes.

In accordance with professional standards and codes of ethics for the various practitioners and clinicians who perform life care planning, the client (also known as the evaluee; see later) is considered the person with a disability or illness who receives services. In life care planning, the client is defined as the person who is the subject of the life care plan. In the forensic or litigation setting, the individual for whom the life care plan is being prepared is considered the evaluee because the professional involved in life care planning is acting as a consultant rather than one who provides treatment.[20]

Furthermore, the individual with an injury, illness, or impairment is assessed individually with respect to findings reported in the literature. The client is a study unto itself. It is important to apply the individual's specific and unique circumstances to the data and research available in the literature, not the research and data in the literature to the individual. It needs to be understood that the entire person must be examined and compared preinjury and postinjury. Although common approaches and methodologies exist, clinical judgment is required to determine the true effect of injury or illness on an individual.[21]

The following are the goals of a life care plan[19]:

1. To assist the client in achieving optimal outcomes by developing an appropriate plan to prevent complications and to restore function. This may include recommendations for evaluations or treatment that may contribute to the client's level of wellness or provide information regarding treatment requirements.
2. To provide health education to the client and interested parties, when appropriate.
3. To develop accurate and timely cost information and specificity of service allocations easily used by the client and interested parties.
4. To develop options for care that may be necessary for other situations.
5. To communicate the life care plan and its objectives to the client and interested parties, when appropriate.
6. To develop measurement tools used to analyze outcomes.
7. To routinely develop comprehensive assessments of the projected goals of the life care plan, whenever possible.

TRAINING, EDUCATION, AND CERTIFICATION

The life care planner must have skill and knowledge in understanding the health care needs addressed in a life care plan. Consultation with others and obtaining education are expected when the life care planner must address new or unfamiliar health care needs. The life care planner must be able to locate appropriate resources when necessary. The life care planner provides a consistent, objective, and thorough methodology for constructing the life care plan, while relying on appropriate medical and other health-related information, resources, and personal expertise to develop its content. The life care planner relies on state-of-the-art knowledge and resources to develop a life care plan.

Specialized skills are required to successfully develop a life care plan, such as the ability to research, critically analyze data, manage and interpret large volumes of information, attend to details, demonstrate clear and thorough written and verbal communication skills, develop positive relationships, create and use networks for gathering information, work autonomously, and demonstrate a professional demeanor and appearance.

According to the standards of practice developed through the IALCP (revised 2006),[19] the life care planner must

- Possess the appropriate educational requirements as defined by their professional standards (eg, nurses should possess the requirements to acquire licensure, rehabilitation counselors should possess the requisite master's degree, and other health professionals should possess the required degree for their fields).
- Maintain current professional licensure or national board certification within a professional health care discipline.
- Demonstrate completion of an accredited program in nursing or a baccalaureate or higher-level educational program in a professional health care field. Fields may include nursing, rehabilitation counseling, medicine, physical, occupational or speech therapy, and psychology.
- Demonstrate that professional discipline provides sufficient education and training to ensure that the life care planner has an understanding of human

anatomy and physiology, pathophysiology, the health care delivery system, the role and function of various health care professionals, and clinical practice guidelines and standards of care.

- Participate in specific continuing education required to maintain the individual practitioner's licensure or certification within his or her profession.
- Obtain continuing education or training to remain current in the knowledge and skills in the field.

WHO PREPARES LIFE CARE PLANS?

In addition to rehabilitation counselors, allied health professionals (eg, occupational therapists, physical therapists, speech language pathologists, nurses, dietitians, counselors, psychologists, dentists, audiologists, and so forth) also develop projected care based on published formats used in life care planning.[14,16] Although it is important that the various participants have a rehabilitation education and relevant certification in their area of specialty before engaging in the life care planning process, this by itself is insufficient; additional education and experience are necessary.[22,23] A qualified life care planner must be a collaborator, participant, and author of the life care plan.[24]

Seven certifications prevalent in the practice of rehabilitation counseling, life care planning, and case management were researched on the following descriptive variables: inception; financial (profit) status; accreditation[25,26]; eligibility; examination; continuing education requirements; and code of ethics/standards of practice (**Table 1**). Often individuals with one or more of these certifications are involved in preparing a life care plan.

DESCRIPTIONS OF CERTIFICATION PROGRAMS

The descriptive paragraphs that follow are excerpted from the Web sites of various certification accreditation bodies, on which are described the requirements for each type of certification. The reader is encouraged to review the full information for each certification program on the respective Web sites.

Certified Rehabilitation Counselor

The Commission on Rehabilitation Counselor Certification (CRCC) sets the standard for quality rehabilitation counseling services in the U.S. and Canada. As an independent, not-for- profit organization, the CRCC has certified more than 30,000 counselors with its widely recognized Certified Rehabilitation Counselor (CRC) and Canadian Certified Rehabilitation Counselor (CCRC) designations.[27]

Certified Case Manager

Case management is a collaborative process that assesses, plans, implements, coordinates, monitors, and evaluates the options and services required to meet the client's health and human service needs. It is characterized by advocacy, communication, and resource management and promotes quality and cost-effective interventions and outcomes. ... Certification as a Certified Case Manager (CCM) is a voluntary professional credential sponsored by the Commission for Case Manager Certification (CCMC).[28]

Certified Disability Management Specialists

The current Certification of Disability Management Specialists Commission (CDMSC) was established in 1984 as the Certification of Insurance Rehabilitation Specialists

Table 1
Summary of rehabilitation certifications on selected variables

Type of Certification Program	Independent Accreditation	Year Established	Minimum Education Required	Minimum Experience Required	Code of Ethics/ Standards of Practice	Examination Required	CEUs Required	Nonprofit
Certified Rehabilitation Counselor	Yes	1975	Yes	Yes	Yes	Yes	Yes	Yes
Certified Case Manager	Yes	1993	Yes	Yes	Yes	Yes	Yes	Yes
Certified Disability Management Specialist	Yes	1984	Yes	Yes	Yes	Yes	Yes	Yes
Certified Life Care Planner	No	1996	Yes	Yes	Yes	Yes	Yes	No
American Board of Vocational Experts	No	1980	Yes	Yes	Yes	Yes	Yes	Yes
Certified Nurse Life Care Planner	No	1999	Yes	Yes	Yes	Yes	Yes	Yes
Certified Vocational Evaluator	No	1981	Yes	Yes	Yes	Yes	Yes	Yes

Data from Field T, Choppa A, Johnson C, et al. Rules of evidence vs professional certifications: the real basis for establishing admissible testimony by rehabilitation counselors and case managers. Rehabilitation Professional 2007;15:7–16.

Commission; in 1996 the Certification of Insurance Rehabilitation Specialists Commission changed to its name to CDMSC. "The CDMSC is the only nationally accredited and independent organization that certifies disability management specialists. Disability management specialists analyze, prevent and mitigate the human and economic impact of disability for employees and employers ...."[29]

CDMSC's mission is to "advance the field of disability management through the utilization of certified practitioners; evaluate and respond to the trends in disability management; promote continuing education while identifying key strategies, skills, and collaboration to ensure best practices in disability management."[29]

Certified Life Care Planner

At time of original writing, the Web site was not functional on this issue stating "This section of the CHCC website is near completion for updating, but more time is needed. Thank you for your patience." In an e-mail memo sent to "All Members of the life care planning Community," information released indicates that ICHCC in "the Spring of 2002 was restructured to S-Corp for profit," and the NCCA application "is completed, and following final review by the Board of Commissioners within the next few days, it will be made available to you" implying that CHCC will refile the required papers for accreditation.[30]

As of November 15, 2012, however, the following development was noted at the International Commission on Health Certification's Web site:

> We are pleased and excited about our application to the National Commission for Certifying Agencies (NCCA). We are working hard to ensure that your credential remains above and beyond approach and that the ICHCC becomes an accredited agency that is in itself above and beyond question or approach. We have engaged two outside consultants to work with us in preparing the extensive application of the NCCA for review. We have received their input and are now revising out a two-volume application so that the field will have an accredited testing agency by the Fall of 2012.[31]

American Board of Vocational Experts

> The American Board of Vocational Experts is a professional credentialing body established as a not-for-profit organization. Its Diplomats and Fellows have academic preparation in several disciplines (rehabilitation, psychology, economics and various aligned disciplines) and in assessment, counseling and consulting. Prior to completion of the certification process, professionals may be associate or student members of ABVE.[32]

Certified Nurse Life Care Planner

> The American Association of Nurse Life Care Planners Certification Board (AANLCPCB) provides oversight of the certification exam for nurse life care planners. This oversight includes item writing and test development, tracking of certificants, quality assurance of the exam, and update of exam content based on industry changes. A passing score on the certification exam allows a nursing professional to utilize the designation Certified Nurse Life Care Planner (CNLCP). The Certification Board is a voluntary organization comprised of six Registered Nurses specializing in life care planning who have earned the designation of CNLCP as well as one public member with an interest in the field.[33]

The mission of the AANLCP Certification Board "is to promote expertise and professionalism in the nurse life care planning by recognizing practitioners who have met defined qualifications and demonstrated knowledge through a certification examination in the specialty."[33]

Certified Vocational Evaluator

CCWAVES [the Commission on Certification of Work Adjustment and Vocational Evaluation Specialists] is a nationally-recognized certifying body that sets, maintains and promotes high standards consistently and responsively for persons who practice vocational evaluation, work adjustment, and career assessment. Certified Vocational Evaluation Specialist (CVE): Persons who earn the designation of a Certified Vocational Evaluation Specialist (CVE) have demonstrated that they possess at least an acceptable minimum level of knowledge (as determined by the Commission) with regard to the practice of their profession. It is intended to help achieve widespread acceptance of the CVE designation by legislators, employers, consumers, peers, other human service professionals and the general public. The primary purpose of this certification process is to provide assurance that those professionals engaged in vocational evaluation meet acceptable standards of quality. Work in the community is foundational to the practices of vocational evaluation and work adjustment. The absence of work, real or simulated, indicates that the service provided is not vocational evaluation or work adjustment.[34]

The Certified Vocational Evaluator certificate that was available through the Commission on Certification of Work Adjustment and Vocational Evaluation Specialists ended with the dissolution of Commission on Certification of Work Adjustment and Vocational Evaluation Specialists in 2009.[34]

Many life care planners are asked at deposition if they are board certified in this professional specialty. Many explain they are not, then justify why it is not required. Several explain that they have been doing the work for years and do not see the need to complete yet another certification examination. Some portray that being a Certified Rehabilitation Counselor prepares them for life care planning and it is a board certification in rehabilitation (The Council on Rehabilitation Education requires basic life care planning education as part of the master's program in rehabilitation counseling [see standard C-10–12]). Life care planning is a tool of advanced case management, so certification as a case manager may be adequate. Elements of all of these arguments may be true. No state requires that an individual be a Certified Life Care Planner (nor a Certified Rehabilitation Counselor, Certified Case Manager, or Certified Disability Management Specialist, and so forth) to testify as an expert. Moreover, some have criticized that the board for life care planning is a private for-profit organization. Additionally, most people on a jury are familiar with board certification as it relates to medicine, which can serve to increase the credibility of a life care planner.

Other professions have individuals who have elected to be part of the subspecialty of life care planning. Physicians, physical therapists, occupational therapists, speech language pathologists, and psychologists have undergone the requisite training and certification, and follow the standards of practice for life care planning.

Recommendations for life care planners and those who seek to use the services of life care planners include the following[35]:

1. Appropriate education and credentials
2. Knowledgeable about the medical aspect of disability or disabilities
3. Relevant specialized training
4. Belong to and, better yet, are active in appropriate organizations (eg, International Association of Rehabilitation Professionals [IARP], Case Management Society of America, IALCP, and American Association of Nurse Life Care Planners)

5. Life care plans are developed according to established and accepted standards of practice, ethics, and published methodologies
6. Life care plans include proper foundation (including medical)
7. Life care plans include up-to-date and current knowledge within the parameters of the profession
8. Life care planners must be familiar with relevant literature
9. Life care planners must be familiar with the rules of the jurisdictions in which they practice
10. Life care planners must be knowledgeable about applicable Federal Rules of Evidence when testifying in personal injury litigation[36]
11. Life care planners are not scriveners or secretaries, who simply write down whatever someone else recommends; conversely, neither do life care planners know it all
12. Life care planners must stay within their area of expertise or scope of practice
13. Life care planners use all skills and understand the premise in which to coordinate a life care plan
14. The professional should consider certification as a life care planner
15. Life care planners need to be aware of the intangible

LIFE CARE PLAN RESOURCES

The life care planning industry continues to grow, change, and modify the scope of practice for catastrophic case management. The IALCP is well established and publishes the standards of practice. In collaboration with the IARP, these bodies publish the *Journal of Life Care Planning*, an ongoing peer-reviewed journal focusing on issues relevant to life care planning.[37]

The University of Florida, Kaplan College (online training leading to certification), Capital Law School paralegal program, the Institute for Medical-Legal Education, IARP, and many other organizations have been preapproved for training related to obtaining or maintaining certification.[38] The Foundation for Life Care Planning Research has been established and supports doctoral student dissertations and other qualified research efforts.[39] Life care planning summits with endorsements from several organizations have been held biannually since 2000, leading to transdisciplinary and transorganizational consensus on many topics and issues.

Although life care planning principles can be used in almost any aspect of care management, it is particularly useful in complex medical cases because the principles and methods that have been developed provide for needed quality care, reduce errors and omissions, prevent clients from slipping through administrative cracks, and reduce the failure to take into account various aspects that effect the ultimate outcome of the client's medical care.[1,40]

Being up to date on life care planning issues can occur through several means. Attending conferences that feature or have special sessions on life care planning issues (eg, the annual life care planning conference or the IALCP-sponsored conference associated with the IARP Conferences, and participating in the life care planning biennial summits) is one way to obtain continuing education credits specific to life care planning.

Keeping current on developments in life care planning through subscriptions to the *Journal of Life Care Planning*, *Care Management*, *Journal of Forensic Vocational Assessment*, and the *Journal of Rehabilitation* can also provide contemporary education in a variety of related topics.

In addition to staying current, the credible life care planner will have read at least some life care planning–oriented books, booklets, articles, and related information.

Various materials on life care planning and vocational opinions have been published. One of the better-known publications is the *Guide to Rehabilitation* by Deutsch and Sawyer,[2] a title that unfortunately is out of print but may be available in university holdings.

Life Care Planning and Case Management Handbook, edited by Weed and Berens[14] (for disclosure, one of the authors of this article), and *Pediatric Life Care Planning and Case Management*, edited by Riddick-Grisham and Deming,[16] are contemporary resources published by CRC Press. Also published are booklets on life care planning and vocational opinions offered by Elliott & Fitzpatrick.[41] An inventory of potentially helpful publications, a list of almost 200 resources, was published in 2002 in the *Journal of Life Care Planning*.[42]

Many professional associations have Web sites and Listservs and routinely publish information, articles, and news on life care planning. These include the Legal Nurse Consultants group,[43] Care Planners Network,[44] IARP/IALCP,[45] and the Commission on Health Care Certification,[30] all of which offer additional information for life care planning–related professionals.

PHILOSOPHIC OVERVIEW AND BASIS

As a member of a health care profession, the life care planner must remain within the scope of practice for his or her profession as determined by state, provincial, or national bodies. The functions associated with performing life care planning are within the scope of practice for health care professionals or are evidenced by assessment.

Analysis of data and evaluation of care recommendations are key elements in the functions of life care planning. In performing these elements, the life care planner communicates with a variety of health care professionals regarding a case. The life care planner does not assume decision-making responsibility beyond the scope of his or her own professional discipline.

The life care plan has as its basis the scientific principles of medicine and health care. In coordinating a life care plan it is necessary to establish a medical, rehabilitation, case management, or psychological foundation for the items recommended in the life care plan. Five components are used to establish the medical foundation for the life care plan[46]: (1) using the medical records, (2) coordinating with the treatment team, (3) using consulting specialists, (4) using clinical practice guidelines, and (5) using research literature. Similar steps are used in establishing case management foundation, although the current case manager would also be consulted. Establishing a rehabilitation foundation may also include using personal expertise, training, and clinical judgment. A psychological foundation is also established with similar steps as noted previously; however, it may also include coordinating efforts with a psychologist or mental health counselor.

ETHICAL CONSIDERATIONS

The primary goal of practice ethics is to protect clients, provide guidelines for practicing professionals, and enhance the profession as a whole.[19] Within the life care planning specialty practice all practitioners are members of one or more professional disciplines and are licensed or certified. It is expected that life care planners follow appropriate relevant ethical guidelines within their areas of professional practice and expertise. Life care planners are expected to maintain appropriate confidentiality, avoid dual relationships, adequately advise clients of the role of the life care planner, and maintain competency in their profession.

PROCESS

The process of preparing a life care plan typically includes the following procedures[2,8,14]:

- Receiving the referral and obtaining case information
- Reviewing medical records and supporting documentation
- Making initial interview arrangements
- Preparing initial interview materials
- Conducting a clinical interview
- Consulting with therapeutic team members
- Preparing preliminary life care plan opinions
- Filling in the holes with consultations and evaluations
- Researching costs and sources
- Finalizing the life care plan
- Distributing the life care plan

Categories to be considered within a life care plan include the following[2,8,14,16]:

- Projected evaluations
- Projected therapeutic modalities
- Diagnostic testing and educational assessment
- Wheelchair needs
- Wheelchair accessories and maintenance
- Aids for independent functioning (and assistive technology)
- Orthotics and prosthetics
- Home furnishings and accessories
- Drug and supply needs
- Home care and facility care
- Future medical care, routine
- Transportation
- Health and strength maintenance
- Architectural renovations
- Potential complications
- Future medical care and surgical intervention or aggressive treatment
- Orthopedic equipment needs
- Vocational and educational plan

As noted in the IALCP standards of practice, the coordination and preparation of a life care plan involves a multifactorial approach. Life care plans are inclusive of the following processes.

Assessment

Assessment is the process of data collection and analysis involving multiple elements and sources. The life care planner

- Collects data that are systematic, comprehensive, and accurate.
- Collects data about medical, health, biopsychosocial, financial, educational and vocational status, and needs.
- Obtains information from medical records, client, family, or significant others (when available or appropriate), and relevant treating or consulting health care professionals. If access to any source of information is not possible (eg, denied permission to interview the client), this should be so noted in the report.

Plan Development Research

Determining content and the cost of research components of life care planning requires a consistent, valid, and reliable approach to research, data collection, analysis, and planning. The life care planner

- Determines current standards of care and clinical practice guidelines from reliable sources, such as current literature or other published sources, in collaboration with other professionals, education programs, and personal clinical practice.
- Researches options and costs for care, using sources that are reasonably available to the client.
- Considers appropriate criteria for care options, such as admission criteria, treatment indications or contraindications, program goals and outcomes, whether recommended care is consistent with standards of care, duration of care, replacement frequency, ability of the client to appropriately use services and products, and that care is reasonably available.
- Uses a consistent method to determine available choices and costs.
- When available or helpful in providing clarity, uses classification systems (eg, International Classification of Diseases-9, *Current Procedural Terminology*) to correlate care recommendations and costs.
- Maintains knowledge of care standards, services, and products through continuing education, literature, exhibits, and so forth.

Data Analysis

The life care planner analyzes data to determine client needs and consistency of care recommendations with standards of care, and assesses need for further evaluations or expert opinions.

Planning

This requires the life care planner to follow a consistent method for organizing data, create a narrative life care plan report and cost projections, develop and use written documentation tools for reports and cost projections, and develop recommendations for content of the life care plan cost projections for each client and a method for validating inclusion or exclusion of content.

Collaboration

The life care planner develops positive relationships with all parties, seeks expert opinions as needed, and shares relevant information to aid in formulating recommendations and opinions.

Facilitation

The life care planner maintains objectivity and assists others in resolving disagreements about appropriate content for the life care plan, and provides information about the life care planning process to involved parties to elicit cooperative participation.

Evaluation

The life care planner reviews and revises the life care plan for internal consistency and completeness, reviews the life care plan for consistency with standards of care and seeks resolution of inconsistencies, and provides follow-up consultation to ensure that the life care plan is understood and properly interpreted.

Testimony

If the life care planner engages in practice that includes participation in legal matters, the life care planner acts as a consultant to legal proceedings related to determining care needs and costs, may provide expert sworn testimony regarding development and content of the life care plan, and maintains records of research and supporting documentation for content of the life care plan.

Life care planning research continues to increase in depth, breadth, and sophistication, with an eye toward underscoring reliability and validity criteria and enhancing the standards of practice.

SUMMARY

Life care planning has emerged as an effective method to predict future care needs and costs. The specialty practice continues to grow and develop new horizons. It is of specific importance that a coordinated effort with standardized approaches be promoted to ensure that the industry as a whole progresses and becomes more effective. As more professionals, including allied health professionals, become involved in this process, the practice will mature and develop more effective outcome measurements. Some universities are developing doctoral programs to endorse or encompass life care planning procedures and methods. A 2003 unpublished study of accredited graduate rehabilitation counselor training programs revealed that two-thirds offer training in life care planning.[47] The Commission on Rehabilitation Education accreditation requires some content related to life care planning within its curriculum.[48] In civil litigation, defense attorneys have increasingly turned to rehabilitation professionals to consult on life care planning issues. It is incumbent on the rehabilitation professional to ensure that services offered are consistent with the standards of the industry. Building on the work of others, rather than reinventing the wheel, assists in achieving this goal.

REFERENCES

1. Weed R, Riddick S. Life care plans as a case management tool. Individual Case Manager Journal 1992;3(1):26–35.
2. Deutsch PM, Sawyer HW. Guide to rehabilitation. White Plains (NY): Ahab Press; 1985.
3. Zasler N. A physiatric perspective on life care planning. The Rehabilitation Professional 1994;9:57–61.
4. Choppa A, Johnson C, Shafer LK, et al. The efficacy of professional clinical judgment: developing expert testimony in cases involving vocational rehabilitation and care planning issues. J Life Care Plan 2004;3(3):131–50.
5. Deutsch P. Life care planning: into the future. Journal Private Sector Rehabilitation 1994;9:79–84.
6. McGowan J, Porter T. An introduction to the vocational rehabilitation process. Washington, DC: US Department of Health, Education and Welfare; 1967.
7. Weed R, Field T. The rehabilitation consultant's handbook. 3rd edition. Athens (GA): Elliott & Fitzpatrick; 2001.
8. Deutsch PM, Raffa F. Damages in tort action, vols. 8 and 9. Albany (NY): Matthew Bender; 1981.
9. Blackwell T, Kitchen J, Thomas R. Life care planning for the spinal cord injured. Athens (GA): Elliott & Fitzpatrick; 1997.
10. Deutsch P, Weed R, Kitchen J, et al. Life care plans for the head injured: a step by step guide. Athens (GA): Elliott & Fitzpatrick; 1989.

11. Deutsch P, Weed R, Kitchen J, et al. Life care plans for the spinal cord injured: a step by step guide. Athens (GA): Elliott & Fitzpatrick; 1989.
12. Kitchen J, Cody L, Deutsch P. Life care plans for the brain damaged baby: a step by step guide. Orlando (FL): Paul M. Deutsch Press; 1989.
13. Weed R, Sluis A. Life care plans for the amputee: a step by step guide. Boca Raton (FL): CRC Press; 1990.
14. Weed R, Berens D, editors. Life care planning and case management handbook. 3rd edition. Boca Raton (FL): St. Lucie/CRC Press; 2010.
15. Riddick S, Weed R. The life care planning process for managing catastrophically impaired patients. In: Bancett S, Flarey D, editors. Case studies in nursing case management. Gaithersburg (MD):: Aspen Publishers; 1996. p. 61–91.
16. Riddick-Grisham S, Deming L. Pediatric life care planning and case management. 2nd edition. Boca Raton (FL): CRC Press; 2011.
17. Field T, Choppa A. Admissible testimony: a content analysis of selected cases involving vocational experts with a revised clinical model for developing opinion. Athens (GA): Elliott & Fitzpatrick; 2005.
18. Weed R, Berens D. Life care planning after TBI: clinical and forensic issues. In: Brain injury rehabilitation. 2nd edition. New York: Demos Medical Publishing; 2012.
19. International Academy of Life Care Planners. Standards of practice for life care planners. J Life Care Plan 2006;5(3):123–9.
20. Barros-Bailey M, Carlisle J, Graham M, et al. Who is the client in forensics? Journal Forensic Vocational Analysis 2009;12(1):31–4.
21. Choppa A, Johnson C. Response to estimating earning capacity: venues, factors and methods. Estimating Earning Capacity: A Journal of Debate and Discussion 2008;1(1):41–2.
22. Weed R. Life care planning questions and answers. Life Care Facts 1989;1:5–6.
23. Weed R. Comments regarding life care planning for young children with brain injuries. Neuro Law Letter 1997;6:112.
24. Weed R. The life care planner: secretary, know-it-all, or general contractor? One person's perspective. J Life Care Plan 2002;1:473–7.
25. National Organization for Competency Assurance, National Commission for Certifying Agencies. Standards for the accreditation of certifying programs (2004, rev). Washington, DC: National Organization for Competency Assurance; 2004.
26. Field T, Choppa A, Johnson C, et al. Rules of evidence vs. professional certifications: the real basis for establishing admissible testimony by rehabilitation counselors and case managers. Rehabilitation Professional 2007;15:7–16.
27. Commission on Rehabilitation Counselor Certification. Certified rehabilitation counselor. Available at: www.crccertification.com. Accessed July 19, 2012.
28. Weed R, Berens D. Life care planning after TBI: Clinical and forensic issues. In: Zasler N, Katz D, Zafonte R, editors. Brain injury rehabilitation. 2nd edition. New York (NY): Demos Medical Publishing. p.1437–53.
29. Certified Disability Management Specialist. Available at: www.cdms.org. Accessed July 19, 2012.
30. Certified Life Care Planner. Available at: www.ichcc.org. Accessed July 19, 2012.
31. ICHCC Accreditation. International Commission of Health Certification. Available at: www.ichcc.org/accreditation.html. Accessed November 15, 2012.
32. American Board of Vocational Experts. Available at: www.abve.net. Accessed July 19, 2012.
33. Certified Nurse Life Care Planner. Available at: www.aanlcp.org. Accessed July 19, 2012.

34. Commission on Certification of Work Adjustment and Vocational Evaluation Specialists. Available at: www.vewaa.com. Accessed July 19, 2012.
35. Weed R, Johnson C. Life care planning in light of Daubert and Kumho. Athens (GA): Elliott & Fitzpatrick; 2006.
36. Field T. Vocational expert testimony: what we have learned during the post-Daubert. Journal Forensic Vocational Analysis 2006;9(1):7–18.
37. Journal of Life Care Planning. Available at: www.rehabpro.org/sections/ialcp. Accessed July 19, 2012.
38. Caragonne P. An overview of the field of life care planning: a comparison of training venues, certification processes, current training needs and a guide to life care planning development. The Earnings Analyst 2004;6:63–114.
39. Foundation for Life Care Planning Research. Available at: www.flcpr.org. Accessed July 19, 2012.
40. Weed R. Life care plans as a managed care tool. Med Interface 1995;8:111–8.
41. Elliott & Fitzpatrick. Available at: www.elliottfitzpatrick.com. Accessed July 19, 2012.
42. Weed R, Berens D, Deutsch PM. The bibliography of life care planning and related publications. J Life Care Plan 2002;1(1):73–84.
43. American Association of Legal Nurse Consultants. Available at: www.aalnc.org. Accessed July 19, 2012.
44. Care Planners Network. Available at: www.careplanners.net. Accessed July 19, 2012.
45. International Association of Rehabilitation Professionals. Available at: www.rehabpro.org. Accessed July 19, 2012.
46. Johnson C, Deutsch P, Riddick-Grisham S, et al. Building foundations in life care planning, (standards of practice in life care planning and cases where LCP opinions have been challenged. Presented at the International Symposium of Life Care Planning. Chicago, September 25, 2009.
47. Isom R, Marini I, Reid C. Life care planning: rehabilitation education curricula and faculty needs. J Life Care Plan 2003;2(3):171–4.
48. Commission on Rehabilitation Education. Accreditation manual for masters level rehabilitation counselor education programs. Available at: http://www.core-rehab.org/Files/Doc/PDF/COREStandardsPrograms.pdf%20Standard%20C-10-12. Accessed July 19, 2012.

The Person with a Spinal Cord Injury
An Evolving Prototype for Life Care Planning

Steven A. Stiens, MD, MS[a,b,c,d,*],
Heidi L. Fawber, MEd, LPC, CRC, CCM, CLCP[e,f],
Steven A. Yuhas, MEd, CRC, CLCP, CCM, NCC, CBIS[f,g]

KEYWORDS

- Spinal cord injury • Life care plan • Problem list • Patient-centered care
- Cost of care • Outcome • Prevention

KEY POINTS

- The segmental design of the body permits spinal cord injury (SCI) assessment to be quantitative, repeatable, and predictive of self-care capabilities and assistance required.
- The variety of neurogenic organ impairments resulting from SCI compromise function and complicate health. A variety of published responsive clinical practice guidelines provide peer-reviewed consensus on effective rehabilitation and preventive medicine.
- The design of an SCI problem list that addresses impairments, activity limitations, and barriers to participation provides an ordered spectrum of areas for intervention that translate well into life care plan development and coordinated patient care.
- Life care planning for SCI is a method that produces a living document that can guide care by organizing patient needs into practical categories and useful schedules.
- Life care planning designs and implements systematic prevention of otherwise inevitable complications of SCI to maximize health and minimize eventual care requirements.
- Patients and communities benefit from life care planning by bringing patients with SCI to maximal capability for contribution to family, occupation, and society.

Funding Sources: Lou and Virginia Muhlhofer, Cincinnati, OH, USA.
Conflict of Interest: None to disclose.
[a] Department Rehabilitation Medicine, University of Washington, PO Box 356490, Health Sciences Building, 1959 North East Pacific, Seattle, WA 98195, USA; [b] Spinal Cord Medicine, 2001-2012, University of Washington, PO Box 356490, Health Sciences Building, 1959 North East Pacific, Seattle, WA 98195, USA; [c] Spinal Cord Injury Unit, VA Puget Sound Health Care System, University Hospital, PO Box 356490, Health Sciences Building, 1959 North East Pacific, Seattle, WA 98195, USA; [d] Model Systems in Spinal Cord Injury, University of Washington, PO Box 356490, Health Sciences Building, University of Washington, 1959 North East Pacific, Seattle, WA 98195, USA; [e] Rehabilitation Consultant, PO Box 299, Mars, PA 16046, USA; [f] International Academy of Life Care Planners Section, International Association of Rehabilitation Professionals, Glenview, IL 60025, USA; [g] The Directions Group, Inc, 999 Lake Hunter Circle, Suite A, Mount Pleasant, SC 29464, USA
* Corresponding author. VA Puget Sound Health Care System, University Hospital, PO Box 356490, Health Sciences Building, 1959 North East Pacific, Seattle, WA 98195.
E-mail address: Steven.Stiens@va.gov

Phys Med Rehabil Clin N Am 24 (2013) 419–444
http://dx.doi.org/10.1016/j.pmr.2013.03.006
1047-9651/13/$ – see front matter Published by Elsevier Inc.

INTRODUCTION: THE ANATOMIC INJURY DETERMINES DYSFUNCTION AND LIFE CARE PLAN DESIGN

Life care planning has been established as a methodology for documenting, funding, and orchestrating services, supplies, and opportunities for persons with spinal cord injury (SCI). If implemented prospectively in care coordination, patients with SCI will be most functional, avoid most complications, and achieve their personal potential across their life spans. The International Academy of Life Care Planners has defined a life care plan as a dynamic document based on published standards of practice, comprehensive assessment, data analysis, and research, which provides an organized, concise plan for current and future needs, with associated costs, for individuals who have experienced catastrophic injury or have chronic health care needs.[1] The patient with spinal cord injury provides a prototype for life care planning because SCI produces quantifiable impairments in sensation and strength along with predictable functional outcomes, and responds to a variety of effective interventions recommended by clinical practice guidelines.

Most functions of the spinal cord as a conduit and relay center for sensory and motor signals are well known and understood. As vertebrates, humans have spinal columns consisting of a stack of weight-bearing vertebral bodies, each representing a body segment. These segments have evolved with a spectrum of functional specializations, such as structures as simple and essential as rib and intercostal muscles for ventilation or as complicated as the upper extremity positions of the hand for fine movements. Spinal cord lesions, therefore, most predictably interrupt function at segments that are injured and segments below them. It is the fragility of the spinal cord and the segmental design of vertebrates that presents the opportunity to systematically examine each dermatome and myotomal segment, thus to determine a spinal cord level. That level is predictive through measurement of multiple domains of outcome of functional independence and burden of care.[2]

SCI disrupts the coordination of other body systems by the nervous system, resulting in various organ dysfunctions. These dysfunctions are systematically addressed in the clinical practice of spinal cord medicine through diagnosis, therapy, rehabilitation, caregiving, and self-care accommodations. These methods have been critically analyzed and formulated into SCI guidelines, and over the last decade a variety of clinical practice guidelines have been developed, based on scientific evidence from clinical studies and consensus of expert clinicians' opinions.[3]

In 1995, the American Board of Medical Specialties established the subspecialty of spinal cord medicine, a new branch of medical science that has grown to more than 600 board-certified physicians and for which 15 fellowship training programs are available at academic medical centers throughout the United States. The body of knowledge used to treat the clinical condition and disablement from SCI has been assembled into textbooks that have been recently updated.[4–6] These and other developments have all contributed to the validity of life care plans, and have allowed expert practitioners to deliver prospective care guided by patient-centered life care plans. Life care planning can be a useful tool after SCI, because of the patient's longevity after injury and the complexity of preventive and supportive care needed following the injury. Efficient and economical care plans can provide a template to enable patients in relationships, work, and community service without compromising patient care needs. Persons with SCI have been the early and ongoing subjects of life care plans that have been proved to be effective for decades. These individuals exemplify the impact of designing these plans to quantify the personal and economic consequences.

SCI is one of the more recognizable and understandable chronic conditions. As a prototype subject of comprehensive medical rehabilitation, the published standards of practice that substantiate the validity of accurately formulated and designed life care plans have been continuously refined. The constantly developing field of spinal cord medicine benefits this subspecialty and all the organizations that unite the efforts of rehabilitation professionals.[7]

The scope of this article prevents explication of all qualifications required of life care planners to project the needs of persons with SCI and the full methodology to develop a life care plan for patients with SCI. Resources in the form of Web sites, book chapters, and textbooks that detail the process of SCI life care planning are readily available.[8] Contemporary academic practice in spinal cord medicine brings together collaborative interdisciplinary teams for patient care and research. Clinical care, as well as academic inquiry, includes the perspectives of patients with SCI to reconcile classic literature findings and current practice with new discoveries, recent technologies approved by the Food and Drug Administration, and emerging treatment options under investigation at the basic science or human trial stage. Patients with SCI have continually sought clinical evidence to support treatments and health maintenance care that can be scientifically substantiated for clinician compliance and health insurance coverage.[3] In addition, consumers of health care and adaptive products have developed a culture of the lived experience of disablement with SCI.[9] As life care planners are assessing the needs of patients with SCI, they need to be aware of clinical practice guidelines and current textbooks in the field to ensure that published recommendations guide life care plan designs.

THE ASIA EXAMINATION: DETERMINING SPINAL CORD IMPAIRMENTS

Comprehensive assessment in spinal cord medicine seeks to capture the disablement predicament of each unique person who has an SCI. This process starts with the most recognizable and clinically applicable method for assessing somatic motor and sensory impairment: assessment using the American Spinal Injury Association's medicine examination (ASIA examination), which was updated in 2011.[6] The most fundamental expression of a patient's spinal cord sensory and motor dysfunction can be summarized by the neurologic level of injury (NLI) and the ASIA Impairment Scale (AIS). The NLI is the most caudal normal functioning spinal cord segment demonstrated by bilateral normal sensation and motor strength. The AIS summarizes the functional significance by segregating patients with SCI into 5 categories, A through E. These categories span from complete injury (A), through sensory sparing (B), to motor sparring (C) and functional motor recovery (D), to full recovery (E). The results of an ASIA examination provide functional information that can be predictive of patient performance in mobility and activities of daily living. Although the results are primarily in the impairment domain, patient outcome performance also depends on other domains of disablement, such as activity limitations and participation.[2] The AIS was adapted from the classification scheme designed by Frankel and colleagues,[10] which abstracts findings from the neurologic examination to summarize the degree of somatic sensory and motor impairment.

When combined with the spinal cord level, the AIS provides an estimate of functional outcomes that may be expected with the successful completion of rehabilitation. The Consortium for Spinal Cord Medicine Clinical Practice Guidelines for outcomes provides an in-depth description of the expected capabilities, and therefore estimates the care needs that various people with SCI may have.[11]

PATTERNS OF IMPAIRMENT AFTER SCI: SPINAL CORD SYNDROMES

An SCI is any damage to the structure of the spinal cord that extends from the brainstem at the foramen magnum to the L1 vertebral level, and continues as the cauda equina to distribute final segmental branches to the sacrum and coccyx. Spinal cord tissue consists of external white matter with myelinated ascending sensory and descending motor fibers that cover a core of gray matter containing cell bodies and interconnecting dendrites and axons from interneurons. Insults come from traumatic contusions, disc herniations, hematomas, abscess compressions, ischemic hypoperfusion, and inflammatory destruction.

Neurologic damage can affect any part of the spinal cord, including the multiple nerve roots that descend from the conus. Localized injuries damaging particular segmental levels produce various patterns of weakness and sensory loss. The distinction between upper motor neuron and lower motor neuron injury can be determined anatomically with magnetic resonance imaging (MRI) or with findings from a neurologic examination. An upper motor neuron injury damages the motor nerves with cell bodies in the cortex and axons that travel down the spinal cord to synapse with the lower motor neurons in the anterior horn at the various levels of the spinal cord. A lower motor neuron injury damages the motor neuron cell bodies in the anterior horn or their axons as they traverse the spinal canal and exit at neural foramina below the vertebra that define the spinal level. SCIs are either complete or incomplete for sensory and motor function. Sensory complete is the absence of perceived deep anal pressure in the rectum. Motor complete is the absence of voluntary anal sphincter contraction. Each of these potential insults can produce a variety of pathologic lesions that manifest clinically as distinctive patterns of motor and sensory impairment. The extent of motor and sensory impairment can be quantified by accurately completing the ASIA examination.

Brown-Séquard syndrome results from a lateral hemitransection, lateral compression, or asymmetric contusion of the spinal cord, causing weakness on the side of the injury and ipsilateral, or opposite-sided, loss of pain and temperature sensation by interrupting the crossed spinothalamic tract. Such patients commonly can walk with a cane and an ankle-foot orthosis (AFO). The prognosis for motor recovery is very good over a 3- to 5-month time frame, because of spared descending motor fibers opposite the lesion and motor fibers that cross from one side of the spinal cord to the other. Cauda equina syndrome is caused by compression of multiple spinal roots in the central canal inferior to the conus, which is typically near the L1 vertebra level. A central lumbar disk that protrudes posteriorly is a common cause. Neurologic examination of patients with complete cauda equina injuries show hyporeflexia and muscle wasting in affected myotomes. Symptoms may include unilateral or bilateral lower extremity pain that radiates below the knees and progresses rapidly to produce bowel and bladder incontinence. Any mass in the lumbar or sacral spinal canal, such as a tumor, hematoma, or abscess, can cause cauda equina compression. The prognosis is good, with swift diagnosis through imaging and emergent surgical decompression. Conus medullaris syndrome can result from damage to the conus by compression or ischemia. Typically the gray matter containing the lower motor neurons controlling the pelvic floor is compromised. Findings on examination include an insensate flaccid anal canal and absence of phasic stretch reflex. These patterns of sensory and motor impairments and functional sparring can implicate lesions of various parts of the spinal cord in cross section.

REHABILITATION FOR PATIENTS WITH SCI: IDENTIFICATION OF PROBLEMS AND GOALS

The rehabilitative care of the person with an SCI begins by developing an understanding of the patient's life activity, relationships, and goals in life before the injury.

Rehabilitation is a continuous process to develop a person to her or his fullest physical, psychological, social, educational, and vocational potential. This development is accomplished by eliminating or compensating for any biochemical imbalance, pathophysiology, anatomic impairment, activity limitation, or environmental barrier.[12,13]

This initial and ongoing rehabilitation plan becomes the basis for the comprehensive life care plan. The life care planner is challenged to present an understanding of the patient as a person and extract all of his or her medical needs from the record. The subjective portions of the notes provide valuable information about patient attitudes and compliance with the treatments offered. These windows into the patient's personality are helpful to the life care planner in designing questions and the style in which information is gathered during interviews with the patient and family. The interdisciplinary team is able to formulate a problem list and a plan with short-term and long-term goals.[12] A rehabilitation plan is formulated based on level of injury, patient performance in therapy, associated diagnoses, and complications. Early medical complications encountered include hypotension, pressure ulcers, autonomic dysreflexia, heterotopic ossification, and deep vein thrombosis.[13]

PROBLEM-ORIENTED CHART REVIEW: IDENTIFICATION OF NEEDS AND ORGANIZATION PLANNING

The problem list and established goals (**Table 1**) cue the life care planner when reviewing the patient's medical chart and when conducting needs assessment during preliminary data collection. The problem list is used because the challenge of life care planning is to extract the data required to prepare the best plan using standard life care planning methods. The most useful life care plan can be reconstructed into problem-based interventions for continued care of the patient and for future case management. Review of medical records can be a formidable challenge for the life care planner. The method used by physiatrists serves to recognize and formulate problems, document them in a problem list, review contributions to most specifically define a problem, and determine a next-step diagnostic or treatment protocol as needed.[13]

The first set of problems can best be defined by the medical and surgical diagnoses. An SCI is neurologically classified using the international standards originally developed by the ASIA in 1982 and recently revised in 2011.[6] The first problem is the SCI, which is defined by results from the ASIA examination and summarized by the NLI, AIS, the mechanism for the SCI (such as a motor vehicle accident), and its date. The next problem is spine stability, which refers to the original fracture or dislocation that leads to the SCI and the surgical correction done to reestablish alignments. Information that needs to be captured includes the vertebral levels fused, brace stabilization required, and restrictions in activity.

This section of the problems list also contains previous diagnoses and other complications that are as unique as any patient. The challenge for the life care planner, with the help of the supporting clinician, is to develop a simple and practical outpatient plan for each problem. Nutrition is a critical area of intervention after SCI that benefits from clinical research design. A recent review of nutrition and metabolic response of patients during the first few months after injury confirmed that there is an obligatory weight loss and a reduction in protein stores, with a decline in prealbumin, albumin, and transferrin.[14] Patients recover from the weight loss but need to learn that in the chronic state of SCI, reduced basal energy expenditure can result from the gradual loss of muscle mass. As people with SCI live longer, they are at increased risk at earlier ages for chronic diseases, such as diabetes, osteoporosis, cardiovascular disease, and cerebrovascular disease. The treating clinician is most successful when risk-factor

Table 1
Problem list

Generic Problems	Categories
Problem Group #1: Medical and Surgical	
SCI level, neurologic level of injury	ASIA impairment scale Neurologic level of injury Magnetic resonance imaging of spinal cord contusions—segments affected
Spine stability	Spinal fracture Dislocation Fusion levels—anterior and/or posterior fixation
Diagnoses	Group by body system Specify severity or stage
Nutrition	Weight, body mass index Vitamin deficiencies B_{12}, D_3, zinc
Problem Group #2: Organ-Level Impairments	
Neurogenic skin	Current pressure ulcers Past pressure ulcers and treatment Past flap closures
Neurogenic bowel Neurogenic bladder Sexuality/fertility	Upper motor neuron Lower motor neuron
Problem Group #3: Whole Person	
Mobility	Transfer method Ambulation Wheelchair type
Activity	Range of motion Standing Walking Aerobics
Activities of daily living	Independent vs assisted
Problem Group #4: Participation	
Architectural accessibility Psychological adaptation	Ramps, doors, bathroom, custom Renovations Attitude, mood
Social role function	People in household
Community reintegration	Access Volunteering
Transportation	Public transportation Assisted driver Adapted driver

(continued on next page)

Table 1 (continued)	
Generic Problems	**Categories**
Vocational rehabilitation	Education
	Work history
	Goal identification
	Work trial
Spiritual access	Spiritual tradition, local church

This generic SCI problem list typically applies to most patients with SCI. A problem list includes areas of inquiry or surveillance needed for ongoing spinal level care. Under Generic Problems, categories are listed starting with the SCI level and continue with other diagnoses, impairments, activity limitations, and barriers to participation. Under Subcategories, associated individual characteristics are listed that can be included in the problem list to individualize the problem for the specific patient. Other commonly included problems are pain (neuropathic, myofascial, or arthritic) and substance abuse (alcohol and drugs). The rehabilitation problem list for a patient with SCI starts with the ASIA examination summary as the neurologic level of injury, the cause, and magnetic resonance imaging evidence of spinal cord tissue damage. Spine stability is listed separately with a phrase to describe the procedure and fixation hardware. Thereafter, all other diagnoses requiring treatment or surveillance are listed. Therefore, impairments such as neurogenic bowel and bladder are listed and specified as upper motor neuron or lower motor neuron as reflex activity reveals. The next section of the problem list specifies key activity limitation areas such as mobility and activities of daily living. The patient's personal perception and response to the situation are addressed under the problem psychological adaptation, which addresses patient cognitions and behaviors in response to SCI. Social role function addresses patient relationships with spouse, family, and chosen friends, including responsibilities and emotional need fulfillment. Architectural accessibility covers access and function inside the home, inside buildings, and outside the home. Community reintegration is an effort to maintain or establish life-enriching relationships with friends, businesses, and resources outside the home and on the Internet using social and other media. Vocational rehabilitation is listed for patients that may have the potential to return to volunteer work or employment, which may require retraining or advanced education. Spiritual access is a problem listed if intervention is required to fully reestablish full participation in a life of active faith.

Data from Stiens SA, O'Young B, Young MA. Person-centered rehabilitation: Interdisciplinary intervention to enhance patient enablement. In: O'Young B, Young M, Stiens S, editors. Physical medicine and rehabilitation secrets. 3rd edition. Philadelphia: Hanley & Belfus; 2008. p. 118–25.

reduction is built into patient diets, activity, and medications, and when the life care plan is designed to sustain these efforts in the community.[15]

The next set of problems focus on impairments in organ function. Neurogenic skin is often listed in this problem cluster, and refers to the impairment in sensation and autoregulation of blood flow to the skin below the NLI. For neurogenic bladder, the foremost goals are the protection of renal function and to achieve continence practically, willful independent drainage, and prevention of infection. A rehabilitation care plan for neurogenic bowel has two main parts: the bowel program and bowel care. The bowel program is the entire plan of care for neurogenic bowel and includes the components: diet, fluids, medication, and bowel care schedule.[16] Bowel care is the process for assisted defecation.[16,17]

The third cluster of problems addresses the patient's capability for tasks as a whole person. Mobility for patients with SCI includes a large variety of issues under one problem. These factors can be conceptualized by picturing the patient recumbent lying supine, then extrapolating to the highest level of mobility that can practically be achieved and maintained with equipment and services in the patient's own community. Activity is a new problem being considered by many physiatrists in contemporary practice. Activity as it pertains to SCI is best defined as repetitive sensory and motor stimulation of the nervous system designed to enhance neuroplastic remodeling, maintain range, and increase muscle mass, endurance, and functional performance. Current treatment protocols at a variety of spinal cord centers provide activity-based restorative therapy in hopes of promoting recovery and keeping the patient maximally fit. Life care planners need to seek physician, therapist, and patient responses to these treatments, and decide with the patient's clinicians what recommendations are appropriate for ongoing treatment as an outpatient, in the patient's home, or at other centers.[18,19] Activities of daily living are self-care focused skills that determine the burden of care required for the assistance or independence of the patient with SCI, and are estimated for various spinal cord levels in the outcome guidelines of the Consortium for Spinal Cord Medicine.[11] At the injury-treatment and outpatient rehabilitation stages, self-care activity is emphasized so that the patient can be discharged and to minimize the need for assistance. Advanced task acquisition will allow the person with SCI to make progress toward recreational and employment goals. Almost no activity occurs without some environmental interaction, which is the substrate as well as the catalyst for personal achievement.

The fourth and final set of problems deals with the capacity of the patient to fully enter into life situations: relationships, the economy, and communities of their choice (education, volunteering, work, spiritual). This aspect is termed participation. Architectural accessibility is the problem area that fundamentally addresses the success achieved by patients in interacting within the entire environment (**Fig. 1**). Architectural accessibility is furthered if all aspects of the patient's environment are reviewed for barriers and solutions. Each environment the patient will occupy needs to be reviewed for functional adaptations.[20] The patient is considered in each position throughout the day, including bed, wheelchair, shower, toilet, all the rooms of the home, the family vehicle, and the office or workplace. The primary goal is for the patient to be functional in the home and to be able to complete a daily care schedule. Psychological adaptation is the process used by all patients to understand SCI and its impact on their lives, and to develop a lifestyle that provides health success and satisfaction. The subjective and objective aspects of this experience have been termed quality of life, which is as difficult to define as it is to measure. Hammell[21] has reviewed the literature and has provided perspectives that have focused outcomes on settings for living and access to meaningful life roles. The life care planner must elicit assessments from the treatment team on current diagnoses and required medications, and plan for psychological therapy as an outpatient.[22,23] Social role function is the problem that addresses the challenges the patient has with full participation within the family, for example as a spouse, mother, father, uncle, aunt, brother, or son. In the community, capabilities need to be enhanced to allow quality function as friend, neighbor, and customer. Success with all other problem areas contributes to success in social roles.

The transition between inpatient and outpatient rehabilitation services is a subject that causes distress, because patients often experience barriers when trying to access services in the community after discharge. These barriers could be surmounted more efficiently with better access to interdisciplinary rehabilitation in outpatient clinics, agency home care, and fieldwork models for services. Transitional rehabilitation models have been used to complete physical rehabilitation in the home and community of the patient's choice by linking to community agencies, training family members, and maintaining physical therapy, occupational therapy, and social work services.[24] Community reintegration is a component of the rehabilitation process that brings the physically and psychologically adapting patient into the nearby landscape to explore life situations that will occur away from home. Patients need to resume visiting businesses such as grocery stores, pharmacies, and physician offices.

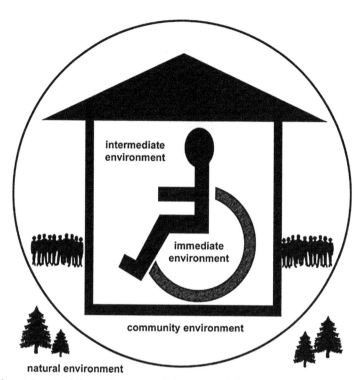

Fig. 1. The patient and the environment. The sectors of the environment should be considered from the patient's perspective. The immediate environment is what is in contact with the person and moves with him or her. The intermediate environment is the space the person occupies that is adapted for him or her. The community environment is the shared space outside of home and work, which has a physical built component and a political component governed by laws. The natural environment is usually minimally adapted and must be accessed with effective mobility equipment or the assistance of others. (*Adapted from* Stiens SA. Personhood, disablement, and mobility technology: personal control of development. In: Gray DB, Quatrano LA, Lieberman ML, editors. Designing and using assistive technology: the human perspective. Baltimore (MD): Paul Brookes; 1998; with permission.)

More importantly, they may wish to frequent restaurants and visit recreational destinations requisite to their passions, which existed before or were refined after the SCI. Long-term adjustment with SCI has been examined prospectively with assessment of the patient's locus of control (perceived control over the events that affect their lives), the environmental barriers and facilitators, and the patient's satisfaction with functional ability. Findings support locus of control as critical to perceived quality of life, productivity status, and satisfaction with performance of activities of daily living. Dominant findings of one study were that social support and peer mentoring were catalysts promoting success, and that stable health and appropriate effective pain management were crucial to subjective satisfaction with community integration.[25]

Transportation can be listed as a separate problem or be included under community reintegration. Exploration of public transportation and preliminary testing for independent driving can often be accomplished during inpatient rehabilitation by certified adaptive driving instructors. A plan for transportation in the life care plan is critical in allowing access to services, education, and work. Success in community transportation is a closely linked prerequisite to success in getting a job.

The life care planner can contribute to success in vocational rehabilitation by recommending adaptive mobility devices with good durability and accurate navigation. Persons with SCI who are in school or gainfully employed report greater adjustment and higher quality of life.[26] The life care plan needs to support patient education needs, adaption equipment, and technology to fully enable employment. There are many unrealized opportunities in work from home, and strong support from the Americans with Disabilities Act (ADA) for accommodations in the workplace.[27] Community travel with public transportation or adapted family vehicles is also an essential goal. Preliminary vocational planning can begin by seeking out the patient's résumé, previous work experience, educational transcripts, and previous vocational assessments. Careful review of patient's past education, recent work history, and job description can come from the vocational counselor, the patient, or the patient's family or employer. Success with self-care, attendant management, community transportation, and independent living are all positive predictors of employment outcomes. Rates of successful vocational interventions after SCI vary from 12% at 1 year to 71% at 2 years of follow-up, with a mean age of 38 years at employment.[28] Careful review of social history will suggest questions for the patient's interview that clarify goals for the life care plan addressing participation in patients' lives. Spiritual access is a problem of importance for various patients because churches are exempt from ADA laws. The goal of fullest participation requires plans for transportation, toilet access, and physical access to the entire building where services are celebrated.

OUTPATIENT REHABILITATION: HEATH MAINTENANCE AND COMMUNITY ADAPTATION

Acute rehabilitation can often rapidly achieve a level of function that plateaus for a period, making a brief intermediary nursing home or group home stay appropriate while adaptations are made to the home. Once discharged to the community, in-home or outpatient therapies are typically initiated. The goals of maximizing function in the home and patient's community may include further family and attendant training. Just as outpatient therapeutic modalities are progressing, the individual with SCI may be faced with funding limitations for ongoing therapy. The life care planner is challenged to identify patient needs and offer innovative programs that maximize outcomes. Contemporary trends in service delivery for exercise are changing, and a variety of centers are emerging in major metropolitan areas that require the attention of the clinicians and life care planners. If a patient with SCI has spared sensation and motor function, repetitive exercises that frequently include assisted functional patterned movement with functional electrical stimulation (FES) can achieve further improvement. In Baltimore, at the International Center for Spinal Cord Injury at Kennedy Krieger Institute, activity-based restorative therapies are being used with SCI patients to prompt remaining nerve cells to contribute to movement while encouraging growth of new nervous system cells. Patients with chronic SCI are assessed and prescribed a variety of weight-bearing and stimulated repetitive exercises that frequently include FES.[29]

The Center for Spinal Cord Injury Recovery, operating as a program at The Rehabilitation Institute of Michigan, also uses nontraditional activity-based therapy programs with innovative exercise systems to optimize the activation of muscles and nerves below the level of injury. This trend to include activity-based therapy at outpatient centers has been emerging over the last decade. These programs may have a role as more persons with SCI are looking for independent exercise programs that can assist them in maintaining their health and fitness. Push to Walk, based in New Jersey, offers an outpatient clinic in which specialty FES equipment is available to clients for either regular training sessions or short-term sessions during which staff teach a program that can be supervised at a local gym or by a privately hired trainer.[30]

The use of FES therapy equipment and other body-weight–supported means of therapeutic ambulation have grown from being available only in rehabilitation facilities to now becoming more common in community-based programs. The goal is physical activity and exercise not only to improve functional status but also to provide health benefits of movement. Programs are also being developed that are considered as independent exercise and health maintenance programs. The Shepherd Center, in Atlanta, Georgia, has opened a community activity-based program, named Beyond Therapy,[31] whose goal is to promote fitness for persons with neurologic injury, improve their health, and reduce secondary complications. Such programs use a wide variety of professional staff and a variety of specialized equipment, such as Lokomat[32] (a robotic therapy-assisted treadmill training system), Restorative Therapies FES rehabilitation therapy equipment, Bioness L300 (electrical stimulation equipment to improve walking functions), Second Step Gait Harness System[33] (a combination walking frame/gait trainer/standing frame), WAVE Vibration Exercise Machines[34] (exercise equipment using vibration training), and Zero G[35] (a harness rail system providing body-weight support while walking), to name but a few.

In the Seattle, Washington area, another similar program known as Pushing Boundaries[30] has experienced trainers who provide range of motion, active assisted range, mat progression of movement, supported standing, FES-driven cycles, and weight-supported treadmill ambulation. FES equipment is not readily available in every community for independent exercise programs; therefore, it is becoming more common for persons to acquire their own exercise equipment, to be used after proper training, from companies such as Restorative Therapies.[36] From the life care planning perspective, such new innovations in SCI rehabilitation, health and fitness programs, and long-term management will need to be closely monitored for the evidence-based value of participation.

LIFE CARE PLANNING: TRANSLATING ONGOING TREATMENT INTO A COMMUNITY-BASED CARE PLAN

Knowing the patient, recognizing needs, and personalizing resources are necessary for the life care planning process to be complete and accurate. To develop the best medical and rehabilitation plan, the patient preferably must be comprehensively assessed at a center by staff with specialized experience in treating SCI patients. The life care plan is a dynamic guide that brings the person-centered rehabilitation plan, patient needs, and preventive services together to proactively guide care (**Table 2**).[37] Knowledge about the person comes from a variety of sources. Subject to availability, photographs, school reports, and transcripts, descriptions by relatives, work histories, and résumés are useful resources to consult.

The life care planning process can start at any time during SCI treatment: acute management, inpatient rehabilitation, or outpatient care. The call for a life care plan most frequently occurs when a patient has reached the outpatient setting. The anticipated needs are best met when a plan is designed after the acute care phase of the SCI. By this time a detailed rehabilitation plan is in place and the patient has had sufficient experience living with SCI to make person-centered choices. Complications are best prevented in situations where the patient is being comprehensively treated at an SCI center with medical cost coverage for indicated services. Current trends have promoted the use of the life care plan in some complex acute care settings to coordinate care for quality, efficiency, and economy. Life care planning principles—assessment,

Table 2
Patient-centered data categories

Preinjury medical history	Pertinent medical problems, surgical history, comorbidities
Personal history	Family overview, social overview, support systems, community overview, social role and responsibilities
Education/training	Educational overview, computer and technology level of knowledge
Vocational history	Vocational overview, dates of employment, employment stability, vocational support system
Military service	Military division, rank, training, length of service, veteran benefits
Postinjury medical history	Level of SCI, ASIA classification, spinal cord syndromes, spine stabilization surgery
Postinjury complications	See **Box 1**. Complications and concerns for SCI
Medical records review—summary	Summary of hospitalizations, surgeries, and operative reports, emergency room visits, diagnostic studies, medications, medical consultations, DME records, medical supply records
Functional abilities	Based on time postinjury and completion of postacute rehabilitation: detailed description of functional strengths and weaknesses, ADLs, IADLs, FIM, mobility, psychological and emotional adjustment, cognitive and behavioral issues, adaptive devices, physical activity and exercise
Attendant care plan	Providers of attendant care, hours of care, agency vs private hire, success vs problems encountered, history of past service providers
Summary—typical day schedule	Detail of average schedule, problems encountered, successes encountered, future goals and desires
Household activities	Preinjury roles and responsibilities, current expectations
Home environment and accessibility	Home description, home owner vs renter, accessibility issues, safety issues, home modification recommendations, home modification and architectural consultation
Transportation	Availability of transportation, type of transportation (own vehicle vs community transport service), driving evaluation and recommendations, recommended vehicle modifications
Community activities	Social support system, community memberships and clubs, church, fitness club
Recreational activities	Sports, adaptive sports access, recreational interests and past participation
Current interdisciplinary team management	Treatment team members, recommendations, need for additional consultants and SCI specialists, access to SCI rehabilitation program, nontraditional professionals
Financial status	Income, health insurance, access to support services
Conclusions	Recommendations, key issues of concern, strengths and weaknesses

The patient-centered data categories provide a structure to distribute information gleaned from chart review and interview. These categories translate easily into the components of the life care plan report.

Abbreviations: ADLs, activities of daily living; DME, durable medical equipment; FIM, functional independence measure; IADLs, instrumental activities of daily living.

research, data analysis, resource identification, and care allocation—have been used in medically complex patients.[38] Early identification of needs clarifies creative alternatives that include consent of family, and collaboration with health insurance and employers to adapt policies and provide accommodations that enable outcomes. As a result, patients can begin to rely on family support, be transported to the best family support, and have alternatives for care in the community with family support.

Various methodologies for the life care planning process have been proposed.[8] The authors emphasize what is best adapted to the patient with an SCI, and note contemporary issues that may enhance success in planning for new cases. The major phases of the life care planning process include needs assessment, plan development, anticipation of complications, the effects of aging, determination of life expectancy, and economic extrapolation based on projected costs.

Needs assessment begins with the medical record review, which includes the diagnoses, secondary functional problems along with the patient's success in therapy, and psychological adjustment to SCI. Needs categories include health (which can be subdivided), mobility, self-care, education, psychosocial issues, housing, transportation, recreation, income, and employment. The chart review method can organize information by problems, as outlined earlier. Plan development requires research and triage of assessments and interventions that can be subdivided into intuitive categories, which can be unique to the life care planner and to particular patients with special needs or aspirations. These categories are called components because they interact to produce the outcome.[39] The patient interview is critical to the authenticity of the life care plan and depends very much on the rapport with the life care planner. This interview complements collaboration with the interdisciplinary team on specific needs assessment. Direct explanation of the benefits of the life care plan engages the patient in the process of life care planning. Inclusion of the closest family member, attendant, or nurse in the interview can be beneficial.

THE COMPONENTS OF THE LIFE CARE PLAN: SPINAL CORD–SPECIFIC CONTENT

The life care planner will wish to address the following topics with the physical medicine and rehabilitation (PM&R) physician and selected members of the interdisciplinary team to develop the life care plan. The following list of life care planning components (**Table 3**) is adapted from Weed's 2004 *Life Care Planning and Case Management Handbook*.[40]

Projected Evaluations

For individuals with SCI, periodic evaluations and reevaluations will be required over their lifetimes. The type of evaluation and its frequency are determined by the level of injury, time after injury, and other associated diagnoses (such as traumatic brain injury and risk factors for coronary artery disease). The traditional allied health professionals who collaborate on inpatient rehabilitation typically continue with outpatient rehabilitation once patients are discharged. After goals are met in outpatient rehabilitation, follow-up consists of an annual evaluation that can be conducted with sequential visits in 1 day or separate outpatient visits with disciplines pertinent to patient needs. An active rehabilitation problem list is maintained, and goals are updated after visits with disciplines pertinent to the case such as spinal cord medicine, rehabilitation nursing, physical therapy, occupational therapy, speech therapy, respiratory therapy, rehabilitation psychology, and recreation therapy. Depending on active goals, the patient may see specialists in nutrition, vocational rehabilitation, urology, or obstetrics and gynecology. Depending on various SCI needs some patients have, specialists

Table 3
Life care plan: components and subcomponents

Life Care Plan Components	Spinal Cord–Specific Subcomponents
Projected evaluations	Annual evaluation: spinal cord medicine physician, physical therapist, speech therapist, occupational therapist, recreational therapist, psychologist, social worker
Projected therapeutic modalities	Physical therapy, occupational therapy, counseling, case management
Diagnostic testing	Laboratory, bone scan, DEXA scans, urodynamic studies, neuropsychological evaluation, educational/vocational evaluation
Wheelchair needs	Power, manual, specialty, shower, recreational
Wheelchair accessories and maintenance	Cushions, trays, lever drive, power-assist wheels, maintenance based on usage
Orthotics	Resting splints, AFOs, KAFOs
Orthopedic equipment needs	Walkers, standing frames, tilt tables
Aids for independent functioning	Environmental controls, adaptive aids, reachers
Home furnishing and accessories	Specialty bed, specialty mattress, lift and track systems, ramps, ventilator equipment, emergency response system, generator
Medication and supplies	Prescriptions, nutraceuticals, respiratory supplies, bowel and bladder supplies, dressings
Home care/facility care	Attendant, home care, residential care, transitional care
Future medical care—routine	PCP, PM&R, orthopedics, urology, pulmonology, psychiatry, other
Future medical care—surgical intervention or aggressive treatment	Wound treatment, plastic surgery, urological procedures, colostomy
Potential complications	Urinary tract infection, pressure ulcer, pneumonia, fracture, syringomyelia
Transportation	Specialty wheelchair van, hand controls, wheelchair vehicle lifts, community transportation services, driver services
Architectural renovations	Ramps, automatic doors, roll-in showers, widened doors
Health maintenance and recreational needs	Adaptive sports equipment, membership fees for recreational groups and sports, adapted exercise equipment
Vocational/educational plan	Educational support costs, counseling, testing, coaching, adaptive resources

Abbreviations: AFO, ankle-foot orthosis; DEXA, dual x-ray absorptiometry; KAFO, knee-ankle-foot orthosis; PCP, primary care physician; PM&R, physical medicine and rehabilitation.

may also include nontraditional interdisciplinary team members such as pharmacists, personal trainers, life coaches, acupuncturists, naturopaths, or massage therapists.

Projected Therapeutic Modalities

The rehabilitation interventions are synergistic because they address various interacting problems with different modalities that work through distinct mechanisms. However, success in each problem produces capabilities that complement success with others. Intermittent focused therapy interventions will frequently be needed over the course of a lifetime of a person with SCI. The need for advanced rehabilitative treatment will be guided by patient-centered goals and performance projection from clinical practice guidelines. Within the first few months after discharge from inpatient rehabilitation, outpatient rehabilitation continues and requires more visits. Over the following year or two, a plan is developed for activity at home and for recreation. Recently discharged patients with new SCI may benefit from independent exercise and intermittent therapy visits to maximize mobility and self-care skills, as well as physical recovery to whatever extent is possible. The range and frequency of therapies may depend very much on resources in the patient's community.

Spinal cord medicine physicians have the perception and experience required to design a lifelong plan for the frequency of rehabilitation modalities necessary over a lifetime, with specifics for patient needs and anticipated complications of SCI. The initial gains in motor recovery and sensation during the first few weeks and months after SCI depend on different mechanisms and present different roles, allowing for continued success with home therapy. Psychological adaptation continues while social roles are redesigned in interaction with family to minimize the impact of aging with SCI, and health maintenance to detect and prevent medical complications. Psychosocial needs, educational level, and other associated factors will influence the need for and potential benefit from well-timed interventions from hospital-based and home care–based therapists and nurses. Neurogenic bowel and bladder management care plans often require modification to meet the demands of dietary changes, different schedules, and home environments.

Diagnostic Testing

The primary care provider and PM&R physician collaborate to determine the need for specific diagnostic testing most appropriate for each individual patient for early and long-term SCI management. These assessments and designs for individual patients are termed disability-related health management and general health promotion.[8] Systems at highest risk include dermatologic, respiratory, gastrointestinal, genitourinary, and musculoskeletal.

Wheelchair Needs/Wheelchair Accessories and Maintenance

The PM&R physician reviews the success patients have with manual wheelchairs in their daily life activity, then consults with physical and occupational therapists to identify the best adaptations or replacements needed to maximize mobility in the home and community environment. Many individuals have access to specialized seating clinics that can allow them to sit in a functional position while preserving skin integrity. Changes in wheelchair prescriptions are driven by changes in skin integrity comfort, propulsion capability, upper extremity overuse, and terrain. Use of a manual wheelchair or a powered one must also be determined as regards which is reasonable, or whether both will be used at different times and places. Occasionally the wheelchair ordered early in rehabilitation is discovered to be less than optimal in regular use in the home community environment, or in a transportation vehicle. Ideally, off-the-shelf adjustable chairs are adjusted and readjusted to optimize the settings, and have a skin-protecting supportive cushion. Patients then demonstrate success in all settings where they will need manual wheelchair mobility. Thereafter, a manual wheelchair is ordered in a fixed or folding frame to meet the demands of the patient's lifestyle. Replacement and maintenance schedules are individualized, based on intensity of use, personal pursuits, and environment. As patients exercise more in their wheelchairs or participate in wheelchair sports, they may require a hand cycle for aerobics, or a rugby or tennis wheelchair.

Aids for Independent Function

A careful review of the occupational therapy and primary nurse notes helps to determine an equipment list for the life care plan. As self-care capabilities improve and evolve at home, review of the patient's daily routine will further refine equipment use and new needs. Review of this list with the occupational therapist will generate ideas for next-step equipment and options for replacement of current equipment. This part of the life care plan can covers a broad range of equipment and devices that enhance function and safety and reduce the physical assistance patients would otherwise require. The devices span the patient's environment from those immediate to them, such as blood pressure and oxygen saturation monitors, lap desks, mouth sticks and reachers, to environmental controls[41] and smart home technology.

Environmental controls can allow persons with severe paralysis, such as those with complete cervical SCI, to increase their level of independent functioning at home, work, and school, or within their general lives. With sip-and-puff and voice-activated environmental controls, even a person with high tetraplegia can independently operate a phone, television, computer, home security system, lights, thermostats, doors, windows, and even more through a computer interface. The computer can be activated by touch, keypad, or even sip-and-puff.[42] In 3 studies of high-level SCI users of electronic aids for daily living (EADLs), Rigby and colleagues[42] noted that the devices used most were the phone, TV, stereo, fan, and lights, and that 94% of 83 EADL users used their devices daily. EADL users reported that the major benefit was increased independence, indirectly improving their feelings of self-worth and self-confidence. Smart home technology has no current consensus definition,[43] but it is generally accepted to include an internal network, intelligent control, and/or home automation with links to services and systems outside the home. The automatic systems can control lighting, temperature, multimedia systems, security, windows, and doors. The goal of assistive technology is not only to increase independence but also to increase independent activity and participation in life functions. Self-driven productivity improves quality of life. The rehabilitation engineer is an essential resource when determining smart home technology and EADL recommendations within the life care plan, given the expense of such specialized technology as well as the wide array of alternatives and resources available in the marketplace.[44]

Orthotics

In SCI rehabilitation and management, bracing and orthoses are commonly prescribed for multiple reasons: improved positioning to decrease the development of contractures (resting splints for upper and lower extremities), to help protect skin and prevent skin breakdown, and to prevent foot drop. Pressure relief ankle-foot orthoses (PRAFOs) and elbow protectors protect and enhance mobility. The PM&R physician will collaborate with the occupational and physical therapists to assist in advising the type of bracing, as well as the need for future bracing replacements and repair. Consultation with an orthotics and prosthetics professional is an invaluable resource when developing appropriate long-term recommendations.

Home Furnishing and Accessories

Within the life care planning process, significant effort should be made to identify installable adaptive equipment, specialized furniture, and architectural modifications for the home, yard, school, and office settings that best enable the person with SCI. These items can reduce attendant care needs, more effectively use space, maximize organization and productivity, and contribute to family life. Many of these items may not be funded by health insurance companies, yet can have a profound impact on function, interaction with family, and productivity at work. This section of the plan includes items such as specialty powered adjustable beds, alternating pressure-distributing mattresses, ramps, automatic doors, overhead installed track lift systems, shower wheelchairs, reserve power generators, and emergency response systems.

Drugs and Supplies

This section of the life care plan can be lengthy, given the often complex medical needs associated with the SCI diagnosis, associated impairments, and other related diagnoses that may interact. The need for many supplies is also common with SCI and can include a complex list of items that can be organized by the impairment problem they support. Bowel and bladder supplies include catheters, leg and bed bags, laxatives, suppositories, gloves, incontinence briefs, under pads, lubricants, and digital stimulators. Pulmonary ventilation equipment and supplies include continuous positive airway pressure and bilevel positive airway pressure machines, humidifiers, ventilators, and suction and insufflation-exsufflation machines. Skin care supplies include pillows, foam blocks, positioning wedges, dressings, emollients, and decompression splints.

Home Care or Facility Care

As home and facility care are the most costly aspect of the life care plan, it becomes essential to include the PM&R physician and the interdisciplinary team in designing recommendations for not only the level of care needed but also the specific care and schedule. Again, an individualized approach must be taken with each person with SCI, considering many factors: level of injury, level of independence, care burden, functional independence measure (FIM) scores, cognitive and intellectual functioning, social, environmental, and psychological issues, medical complications, home accessibility, and ultimately the safety of the individual. If a person with SCI is able to return home to an environment that fully accommodates their level of functioning and needs, the amount and level of care may be dramatically different from that provided for the same person returning to a setting that has minimal physical accommodations. Home modifications, specialty adaptive equipment, and environmental controls are expensive items and are rarely funded by insurance companies. For this reason, the need for personal care is often greater than it might be with optimal environmental supports and adaptations.

Rutherford Owen and Marini[45] surveyed the attendant care plan of 55 adults with SCI who had life care plans. Sixty-seven percent of respondents presettlement depended on unpaid family and friends to provide their personal attendant care. For those whose life care plans resulted in favorable settlements, only 34% continued to receive unpaid personal care by family and friends. In 2009, about 42.1 million family members provided caregiving to an adult with limitations in daily activities of living in the United States.[46] Relying on family and friends as the primary source of attendant care can have inherent problems. It can have a significant effect on the preinjury relationship between the person with SCI and his or her spouse, parent, or significant other. Preinjury roles change to that of caretaker and caregiver. The life care planner must assess the preinjury relationships and support the need for those roles not to be jeopardized. Attendant care services have been found to directly improve reported quality of life of persons with SCI by improving their success in social roles, and access to the community and work.[47]

The rehabilitation physician and life care planner can review personal assistance guidelines for SCI that have been developed by the Paralyzed Veterans of America–sponsored Consortium for Spinal Cord Medicine,[11] which provides guidance on the number of hours of personal care and homemaker assistance needed for different levels of SCI. The life care plan is scheduled by grouping care tasks together and sequencing them during intensive sessions. Many patients have an AM attendant and a PM attendant, and call for emergency needs by cell phone during the day.

The life care plan most commonly provides a person-centered recommendation with the rehabilitation goal of a least-restrictive living option, with return to home being the best option. National Spinal Cord Injury Statistical Center data from 2011 indicate that 88% of persons with SCI are discharged to their preinjury home.[48] However, this is not always possible and it may become necessary for the life care plan to provide temporary alternative living options. Unfortunately, some persons may need to reside in a skilled nursing facility because of the level of their care needs. For example, an SCI patient who uses a ventilator may require a nursing home, group home, or in-home nursing to have ventilatory care. Other medical complications, such as severe pressure ulcers, obesity, and behavioral issues, require specialized nursing care and supervision, as well as emotional support. Family support and availability during the day contribute to limitations that may affect the goal of returning a person with SCI home to the community. If no reliable family support is available, it may also be unreasonable to expect that sufficient hours of reliable attendant care can be obtained, and living alone may not be a safe option for that person.

Future Medical Care: Routine

The PM&R physician can provide insight into the many medical disciplines needed to manage the health of the patient with SCI. Given the impact of SCI on many body systems, a variety of specialists may be needed intermittently over the lifetime of the individual with SCI. The SCI medical guidelines make recommendations for surveillance and prevention of complications common to SCI, and can guide scheduling in the life care plan recommendations.

The primary care provider provides preventive care, surveillance for complications, and nutrition counseling, and helps maintain organ function. The primary care provider receives and organizes the recommendations of other providers and coordinates care to meet patient-centered goals.

The PM&R physician or spinal cord medicine specialist completes the initial rehabilitation, orchestrates goal-focused advanced rehabilitation, and promotes ongoing adjustment to disability, with referrals to other specialists as needed to address complications. These actions include pain management, and recommendations for adaptive equipment and mobility equipment. Urologists who regularly care for a group of SCI patients are consulted as needed to assist the primary care provider and rehabilitation physician in neurogenic bladder management, prevention of frequent urinary tract infection, choice of bladder drainage options (intermittent catheterization/external catheters/indwelling catheter/suprapubic catheter), prevention of bladder cancer, and issues dealing with erection and fertility.

Orthopedists and musculoskeletal medicine specialists provide consultation or brief treatment for varied complications involving the musculoskeletal system, such as spasticity, overuse syndromes, heterotopic ossification, contractures, osteoporosis, and bone fractures.

Gastroenterologists are occasionally consulted for problems with neurogenic bowel management: constipation, diarrhea, fecal impaction, gastroesophageal reflux, and peptic ulcer disease.

Pulmonologists and respiratory therapists provide chronic treatment for broncho-spasms, mucus plugging, pneumonia prevention, expectoration, sleep apnea, and ventilator management.

Other consultants occasionally needed include neurosurgeons to evaluate neuro-logic deterioration, psychiatrists to treat depression, podiatrists to treat foot wounds, and plastic surgeons to close nonhealing pressure ulcers.

By providing effective and efficient medical and health-related professional support systems as well as attendant or nursing services, a comprehensive life care plan should prevent many complications by reducing their frequency, severity, and cost.[49] A comprehensive plan, led by the primary care provider and PM&R specialist, should oversee a lifelong periodic schedule of physician-specialist visits, as needed on the individual SCI case, to help ensure prevention of SCI-related complications.

Transportation

Appropriate transportation options for a person with SCI need to be considered. Access to the community for health care, shopping, citizenship, leisure, and work is essential for the fullest life and contributions. Including transportation in the life care plan may contribute to the effectiveness of the entire plan, as accessible and indepen-dent transportation enables community participation and increases access to care as symptoms and findings emerge.[50] For many with SCI, financial resources may limit options for vehicle modifications. The person with SCI must be considered if the level of injury can be accommodated to allow him or her to drive independently. Regard-less, the person's ability to transition in and out of the vehicle, transition in and out of a wheelchair, and store the wheelchair in the vehicle with or without assistance must be considered. Medical insurance does not routinely cover such modifications. Many individuals with SCI rely on accessible transport services within their community or on others to transfer them in and out of a vehicle that is not otherwise accessible, and to provide their transportation. Driver evaluations and driver training are also needed to assess appropriate equipment and vehicle modifications before purchase. Certified driver rehabilitation specialists provide such specialized services and assist in the best planning for adaptive transportation. After purchase, training will also be required on its safe use. Again, these services are either privately paid for, or may be paid for by workers' compensation, the Veterans Administration, or the state voca-tional rehabilitation system.

Maintenance of Health and Strength

It is important to consider the recreational interests of the person. Adaptive equipment has been designed for a broad array of sports and recreational activities, and many resources are available online, such as the United Spinal Association's TechGuide[51] that provides numerous equipment options. Lifelong, formalized rehabilitation therapy modalities may not be reasonable within the life care plan; however, health mainte-nance is an important consideration for persons with SCI, countering the effects of impaired mobility. The focus is on increasing physical activity, strength, and endur-ance, and to permit the person with SCI to benefit from exercise. The potential benefit of reduced development of medical complications associated with immobility is also considered.

Home Modification/Architectural Considerations

This part of the life care plan is a significant financial aspect, often with limited options for funding. Returning a person to a home environment that is wheelchair accessible and safe is of premier importance. Preliminary home modifications have often been made with the goal of returning the person with SCI to his or her home. These initial modifications may not be optimal or fully completed, and may require later improvements or corrections to initial work. Frequently the person returns to his or her partially modified residence with limited access to the nonmodified remainder of the home. Consultation with professionals familiar with home and building modification is advisable. Occupational therapists experienced with SCI rehabilitation, certified environmental access consultants, and National Association of Home Builders certified aging in place specialists are good resources for recommending appropriate options. Along with the structural and accessibility needs of the home, considerations also include additional space for equipment and supplies, additional space for attendants or caretakers who may remain overnight, and specialty electrical needs for generators, elevators, or other pertinent electrical equipment. Environmental control systems must also be considered as part of the home modification plan, as some technology may reduce the need for certain structural changes.

Future Medical Care/Surgical Interventions or Aggressive Treatment

This section of the SCI life care plan will often include medical services that have been specifically recommended by a treating physician, such as surgical revision to a suprapubic catheter or colostomy for reasons specific to an individual's case. Botox injections for a variety of concerns may also be considered if specifically recommended. Treatment may include surgery because of skin breakdown or plastic surgery to advance the healing process. Rehospitalization for respiratory infection is more common in tetraplegics, and for pressure ulcers in those with paraplegia.[52] A study by Dryden and colleagues[53] revealed that rehospitalizations after traumatic SCI were high in the first 2 years, at the fifth year, and after 10 years. An individual with SCI may also experience chronic medical complications, such as pain or spasticity, for which intrathecal baclofen therapy or spinal cord stimulation may be considered. Additional surgical consideration may include phrenic nerve pacers.

Orthopedic Equipment Needs

SCI cases often include a wide array of orthopedic equipment including walkers, standing frames or tables, tilt tables, and body support equipment. This part of the life care plan is separated from mobility and aids for independent functioning, and reflects purely orthopedic equipment. Replacement of such items must be considered over the lifetime of the person with SCI.

Educational and Vocational Plan

The life care plan may include a section for future educational and vocational training. Educational testing may be included in pediatric or adult SCI cases, depending on educational or retraining goals. For pediatric cases, educational levels and school setting options (public school, cyber school, private licensed school affiliated with a rehabilitation program) may wish to be explored in this part of the life care plan, addressing Public Law 94-142 issues. Private tutoring services, transitional counseling services, vocational counseling services, job coaching, and job placement services may all be included in this part of the life care plan, along with technology (computers or adaptive computer equipment), supplies, and materials (books, journals) related to the academic or vocational plan.

POTENTIAL COMPLICATIONS: POSSIBLE DIAGNOSES ASSOCIATED WITH SCI
Potential Complications

The life care plan will typically provide an overview of potential complications associated with SCI (**Box 1**). Issues such as skin breakdown, infections (urological and respiratory), orthopedic problems (such as overuse syndrome and heterotopic ossification), and psychological complications (depression, adjustment to disability, substance abuse, anxiety, and so forth) are discussed within the narrative report; however, given the limitations in accurately projecting occurrence, frequency, and duration of complications, they are normally not included within the life care plan. Dryden and colleagues[53] studied the use of services after SCI in 233 subjects with matched controls, and found that SCI patients spent 3.3 more days in the hospital, with 47% treated for urinary tract infection, 34% for pneumonia, 28% for depression, and 20% for pressure ulcers as outpatients. Again, the goal of the life care plan is to provide the services and care needed to prevent medical complications.

Potential complications are defined as possible problems rather than probable ones, and their costs are not included in the total cost of the life care plan, presumably because effective life care planning will reduce complications as it provides the structure for quality care.[50] The life care planner will need to carefully document any medical history and/or current complications of an SCI individual if complications in the life care plan are being considered for purposes other than educational. Several serious complications can occur after an SCI, which could be potentially life threatening. Most of these are preventable with proper care an adapted environment and early problem identification.[54,55] Even with the best medical management and selected treatment team, it is essential for the PM&R physician, life care planner, case manager, and others working with an SCI individual to be aware of the multiple complications that can occur. The types of complications and their severity will vary with each SCI individual.

CONCLUSIONS: LIFE CARE PLANS ARE DYNAMIC GUIDES THAT PREVENT COMPLICATION AND ENABLE POTENTIAL

The segmental design of the spinal cord and the standardized systematic ASIA examination allows for an accurate and continuous determination of motor and sensory impairment that complements the FIM used to predict functional outcomes. SCI medicine is a medical specialty that allies with a variety of professions that share an exclusive focus on patients with SCI, which has catalyzed a rapidly developing framework of evidence-based practice. The resulting clinical practice guidelines provide an objective and useful foundation on which to develop life care plans. Ideally the initial life care planning efforts for SCI can begin after the acute phase of injury and rehabilitation, or later as patient decisions and the clinical course have better defined patient-centered needs. At this stage, redetermination of the current SCI level, spine stabilization restrictions, and current and expected medical treatment have been better defined. In incomplete SCI, patient responses to locomotor training and activity-based restorative therapy may decrease costs of care, as outlined in the life care plan.[56] Moreover, the life care plan may be clarified if the person with SCI has returned to the community and has had time to establish a foundation of what medical complications may be of issue, as well as what social, familial, and independent living issues have emerged or have become more challenging. The life care plan can become a resourceful tool for

Box 1
Complications and concerns for SCI (common complications or findings after SCI are included for prevention and recognition)

1. Nervous system
   a. Chronic pain/neurogenic pain
   b. Posttraumatic cystic myelopathy
   c. Posttraumatic syringomyelia
   d. Spasticity
   e. Fatigue/weakness
2. Respiratory system
   a. Pulmonary infection
   b. Pulmonary function
   c. Reduced vital capacity
3. Musculoskeletal system
   a. Upper extremity impairments
   b. Degenerative changes
   c. Fractures
   d. Osteoporosis
   e. Posture problems
   f. Contractures
   g. Heterotopic ossification
4. Cardiovascular system
   a. Autonomic dysreflexia
   b. Deep venous thrombosis
   c. Coronary artery disease
5. Gastrointestinal system
   a. Abdominal pain/abdominal distention
   b. Gastrointestinal hemorrhage
   c. Gastric ulcerations
   d. Ileus
   e. Cholelithiasis
   f. Esophageal problems
   g. Diverticulitis
   h. Hemorrhoids
   i. Fecal impaction
   j. Constipation
   k. Diarrhea
   l. Delayed bowel evacuation
   m. Bowel incontinence

6. Genitourinary system
   a. Urinary tract infection
   b. Bladder cancer
   c. Renal failure
   d. Calculi
   e. Urethral tears
   f. Hydronephrosis
   g. Bladder dilation
   h. Bladder trabeculations
   i. Chronic cystitis
   j. Prostatitis
   k. Epidimyorchidis
7. Skin
   a. Pressure sores
8. Psychosocial function
   a. Adaptation
   b. Adjustment
      i. Apathy
      ii. Anxiety
      iii. Depression
      iv. Social withdrawal/isolation
      v. Suicidal ideation
   c. Self-control/individual choice
   d. Substance use/abuse

proactive interventions to reduce long-term complications and maximize functional well-being, as well as include services, specialized equipment, and home and vehicle modification that were not obtained thus far. In SCI, as in other areas of catastrophic disability, life care planning requires contributions from a wide range of medical and rehabilitation professionals, best specifically experienced in the area of SCI rehabilitation, treatment, and familiarity with potential SCI complications. The foregoing, together with the inclusion of information available through the SCI clinical practice guidelines and input from the SCI patient and his or her family, can help formulate a thorough and accurate life care plan in even the most complex SCI cases.

REFERENCES

1. International Academy of Life Care Planners. Standards of practice. J Life Care Plan 2002;1(1):51.
2. Marino RJ. Domains of outcomes in spinal cord injury for clinical trials to improve function. J Rehabil Res Dev 2007;44(1):113–22.
3. Stripling T, Cohen CJ, Nalle KS. Consortium for spinal cord medicine clinical practice guidelines. In: Lin VW, Bono CM, Cardenas DD, et al, editors. Spinal

cord medicine: principles and practice. 2nd edition. New York: Demos Medical Publishing; 2010. p. 1080–5.

4. Lin VW, Bono C, Cardenas D, et al. Spinal cord medicine: principles and practice. 2nd edition. New York: Demos Medical Publishing; 2010.

5. Campagnolo DI, Kirshblum S, Nash MS, et al. Spinal cord medicine. 2nd edition. Philadelphia: Lippincott Williams & Wilkins; 2011.

6. Kirshblum SC, Waring W, Biering-Sorensen F, et al. Reference for the 2011 revision of the International Standards for Neurological Classification of Spinal Cord Injury. J Spinal Cord Med 2011;34(6):547–54.

7. Academy of Spinal Cord Injury Professionals. Inc. Available at: www.academyscipro.org/. Accessed September 1, 2012.

8. Blackwell TL, Krause JS, Winkler T, et al. Spinal cord injury desk reference: guidelines for life care planning and case management. New York: Demos Medical Publishing; 2001.

9. New Mobility: The magazine for active wheelchair users. Available at: www.newmobility.com/. Accessed September 1, 2012.

10. Frankel HL, Hancock DO, Hyslop G, et al. The value of postural reduction in the initial management of closed injuries of the spine with paraplegia and tetraplegia. Paraplegia 1969;7(3):179–92.

11. Paralyzed Veterans of America. Consortium for Spinal Cord Medicine. Available at: http://www.pva.org/site/c.ajIRK9NJLcJ2E/b.6431479/k.3D9E/Consortium_for_Spinal_Cord_Medicine.htm. Accessed September 1, 2012.

12. Kirshblum SC, Priebe MM, Ho CH, et al. Spinal cord injury medicine. 3. Rehabilitation phase after acute spinal cord injury. Arch Phys Med Rehabil 2007; 88(Suppl 1):S62–70.

13. Stiens SA, O'Young B, Young MA. Person-centered rehabilitation: interdisciplinary intervention to enhance patient enablement. In: O'Young B, Young M, Stiens S, editors. Physical medicine and rehabilitation secrets. 3rd edition. Philadelphia: Hanley & Belfus; 2008. p. 118–25.

14. Thibault-Halman G, Casha S, Singer S, et al. Acute management of nutritional demands after spinal cord injury. J Neurotrauma 2011;28:1497–507.

15. Groah SL, Stiens SA, Gittler MS, et al. Spinal cord injury medicine 5. Preserving wellness and independence of the aging spinal cord injured: a primary care approach for the rehabilitation medicine specialist. Arch Phys Med Rehabil 2002;83(3 Suppl 1):S82–9, S90–8.

16. Stiens SA, Biener Bergman S, Goetz LL. Neurogenic bowel dysfunction after spinal cord injury: clinical evaluation and rehabilitation management. Arch Phys Med Rehabil 1997;78(Suppl 3):S86–102.

17. Pardee C, Bricker D, Rundquist J, et al. Characteristics of neurogenic bowel in spinal cord injury and perceived quality of life. Rehabil Nurs 2012;37(3):128–35.

18. Sadowski CL, McDonald JW. Activity-based restorative therapies: concepts and applications in spinal cord injury-related neurorehabilitation. Dev Disabil Res Rev 2009;15(2):112–6.

19. Edgerton RV, Harkema SJ, Roy RR. Retraining the human spinal cord: exercise interventions to enhance recovery after spinal cord injury. In: Lin VW, Bono CM, Cardenas DD, et al, editors. Spinal cord medicine: principles and practice. 2nd edition. New York: Demos Medical Publishing; 2010. p. 939–50.

20. Stiens SA, Shamberg S, Shamberg A. Environmental barriers: solutions for participation, collaboration, and togetherness. In: O'Young B, Young M, Stiens S, editors. Physical medicine and rehabilitation secrets. 3rd edition. Philadelphia: Hanley & Belfus; 2008. p. 76–86.

21. Hammell KW. Exploring quality of life following high spinal cord injury: a review and critique. Spinal Cord 2004;42(9):491–502.
22. Manns PJ, Chad KE. Components of quality of life for persons with a quadriplegic and paraplegic spinal cord injury. Qual Health Res 2001;11(6):795–811.
23. Boswell BB, Dawson M, Heininger E. Quality of life as defined by adults with spinal cord injuries. J Rehabil 1998;64:27–32.
24. Kendall MB, Ungerer G, Dorsett P. Bridging the gap: transitional rehabilitation services for people with spinal cord injury. Disabil Rehabil 2003;25(7): 1008–15.
25. Boschen KA, Tonack M, Gargaro J. Long-term adjustment and community reintegration following spinal cord injury. Int J Rehabil Res 2003;26(3):157–64.
26. Krause JS, Anson CA. Adjustment after spinal cord injury: relationship to participation in employment or educational activities. Rehabil Couns Bull 1997;40(3): 202–14.
27. Frieden L, Winnegar AJ. Opportunities for research to improve employment for people with spinal cord injuries. Spinal Cord 2012;50(3):379–81.
28. Van Velzen JM, de Groot S, Post MW, et al. Return to work after spinal cord injury: is it related to wheelchair capacity at discharge from clinical rehabilitation? Am J Phys Med Rehabil 2009;88(1):47–56.
29. Kennedy Krieger Institute. Activity-based restorative therapies: concepts and applications in spinal cord injury-related neurorehabilitation. Available at: www.kennedykrieger.org/research-training/biblio/activity-based-restorative-therapies-concepts-and-applications-spinal-cord-. Accessed September 1, 2012.
30. Pushing boundaries. Exercise, health and hope for people with paralysis. Available at: www.pushing-boundaries.com/. Accessed September 1, 2012.
31. Beyond Therapy. A Shepherd Center Program. Available at: www.beyond-therapy.org/. Accessed September 1, 2012.
32. Hocoma. Available at: www.hocoma.com/. Accessed September 1, 2012.
33. Second Step. Helping people walk again. Available at: www.secondstep.com/. Accessed September 1, 2012.
34. WAVE Vibration Exercise Machines. Available at: www.wavexercise.com/index.html. Accessed September 1, 2012.
35. Bioness. Foot drop, drop foot, hand treatment, hand rehabilitation. Available at: www.bioness.com. Accessed September 1, 2012.
36. Restorative Therapies. Holistic techniques that bring you back to balance. Available at: www.restorativetherapies.com/. Accessed September 1, 2012.
37. Deutsch PM, Allison L, Cimino-Ferguson S. Life care planning assessments and their impact on quality of life in spinal cord injury. Top Spinal Cord Inj Rehabil 2005;10(4):135–45.
38. McCollom P. Applying life care planning principles in acute situations. Case Manager 2006;17(5):66–8.
39. Priebe MM, Chiodo AE, Scelza WM, et al. Spinal cord injury medicine. 6. Economic and societal issues in spinal cord injury. Arch Phys Med Rehabil 2007; 88(3 Suppl 1):S84–8.
40. Weed RO, editor. Life care planning and case management handbook. 2nd edition. Boca Raton (FL): CRC Press; 2004.
41. AbleNet. Assistive technology products and specialized curriculum for persons with disabilities. Available at: www.ablenetinc.com/. Accessed September 1, 2012.
42. Rigby P, Ryan S, Joos S, et al. Impact of electronic aids to daily living on the lives of persons with cervical spinal cord injuries. Assist Technol 2005;17(2):89–97.

43. Brandt A, Samuelsson K, Töytäri O, et al. Activity and participation, quality of life and user satisfaction outcomes of environmental control systems and smart home technology: a systematic review. Disabil Rehabil Assist Technol 2011; 6(3):189–206.

44. Downey G. What is a rehab engineer and why do you need one? RehabPro 2007;15(1):33–8.

45. Rutherford Owen T, Marini I. Attendant care and spinal cord injury: usage patterns and perspectives for those with life care plans. J Life Care Plan 2012; 10(4):33–43.

46. Feinberg L, Reinhard SC, Houser A, et al. AARP Public Policy Institute. Valuing the invaluable: 2011 update. The growing contributions and costs of family caregiving. Available at: http://assets.aarp.org/rgcenter/ppi/ltc/i51-caregiving.pdf. Accessed December 30, 2012.

47. Harrell TW, Krause JS. Personal assistance services in patients with SCI: modeling an appropriate level of care in a life care plan. Top Spinal Cord Inj Rehabil 2002;7(4):38–48.

48. Rutherford Owen T, Thomas RL. National spinal cord statistical center cost figures: a comparison to the life care planning approach. J Life Care Plan 2012; 11(2):27–34.

49. Deutch PM, Sawyer HW. A guide to rehabilitation. New York: Matthew Bender; 1993.

50. Weed RO, Berens DE, editors. Life care planning and case management handbook. 3rd edition. Boca Raton (FL): Taylor & Francis Group; 2010.

51. USA TechGuide. Guide to wheelchairs and assistive technology. Available at: www.usatechguide.org/. Accessed September 1, 2012.

52. Cardenas DD, Hoffman JM, Kirshblum S, et al. Etiology and incidence of rehospitalization after traumatic spinal cord injury: a multicenter analysis. Arch Phys Med Rehabil 2004;85(11):1757–63.

53. Dryden DM, Saunders LD, Rowe RH, et al. Utilization of health services following spinal cord injury: a 6-year follow-up study. Spinal Cord 2004;42(9):513–25.

54. Blackwell TL, Weed RO, Powers AS. Life care planning for spinal cord injury: a resource manual for case managers. Athens (GA): Elliott and Fitzpatrick; 1994.

55. Stiens SA. Personhood, disablement, and mobility technology: personal control of development. In: Gray DB, Quatrano LA, Lieberman ML, editors. Designing and using assistive technology: the human perspective. Baltimore (MD): Paul Brookes; 1998. p. 29–49.

56. Morrison SA, Pomeranz JL, Yu N, et al. Life care planning projections for individuals with motor incomplete spinal cord injury before and after locomotor training intervention: a case series. J Neurol Phys Ther 2012;36(3):144–53.

Life Care Planning After Traumatic Brain Injury

Nathan D. Zasler, MD[a,b,]*, Arthur Ameis, BSC, MD, FRCPC, DESS[c,d], Susan N. Riddick-Grisham, RN, BA, CCM, CLCP[e,f,g,h,i]

KEYWORDS

- Traumatic brain injury (TBI) • Life care planning • Physiatry • Medicolegal

KEY POINTS

- A life care plan sets out the full extent of the acquired impairments, likely complications, implications for independence, quality of life, and long-term care needs and then informs the parties about the rationale, including nature, extent, and frequency, for all the goods and services likely to be needed over a person's life span and associated costs.
- Whether from a clinical or litigation perspective, all life care plans should be founded in good science and preferably methodologically sound evidence-based medical practice.
- For patients with traumatic brain injury (TBI), a life care plan requires systematic and thorough consideration of multiple dimensions of central nervous system functioning, including not only the more obvious problems of motor, communication, cognitive, and neuropsychiatric impairment but also other issues, such as pain, fatigue, and psychological responses to trauma, impairment, and disability.
- Some of the major life care plan domains include home and/or facility care, medications, durable medical equipment, and vocational issues. Physicians and life care planners should be aware of common faux pas made in life care plans that can undermine the credibility of a plan as well as a professional's expert testimony.
- Clinicians—physicians or otherwise—involved either in the development of life care plans or in their critique should have a consistent methodology for reviewing the scientific credibility and foundation of such documents.

Funding Sources: None to declare.

Conflict of Interest: None to declare.

[a] Concussion Care Centre of Virginia, Ltd, 3721 Westerre Parkway, Suite B, Richmond, VA 23233, USA; [b] Tree of Life Services, Inc, 3721 Westerre Parkway, Suite B, Richmond, VA 23233, USA; [c] Arthur Ameis Medicine Professional Corporation, 333 Wilson Avenue, Suite 502, Toronto, Ontario M3H 1T2, Canada; [d] Certification Program in Insurance Medicine and MedicoLegal Expertise, Faculty of Medicine, Universite de Montreal, 2900 Boulevard Edouard-Montpetit, Montreal, Quebec H3T 1J4, Canada; [e] The Care Planner Network, 3126 West Cary Street, #137, Richmond, VA 23221, USA; [f] Life Care Manager, 3126 West Cary Street, No. 137, Richmond, VA 23221, USA; [g] Foundation for Life Care Planning Research, 10 Windsormere Way, Suite 400, Oviedo, FL 32764, USA; [h] Sarah Jane Brain Project, 101 West End Avenue, New York, NY 10023, USA; [i] International Association of Rehabilitation Professionals, 1926 Waukegan Road, Suite 1, Glenview, IL 60025-1770, USA

* Corresponding author. Concussion Care Centre of Virginia, Ltd, 3721 Westerre Parkway, Suite B, Richmond, VA 23233.

E-mail address: nzasler@cccv-ltd.com

INTRODUCTION

TBI sequelae typically affect all aspects of a patient's future life: domestic, recreational, vocational, social, and personal. Any good life care plan must accomplish several important goals for a patient with TBI. It must serve to fully and clearly inform all parties to litigation about the rationale, including nature, extent, and frequency, for all the goods and services likely to be needed over a person's life span. It must also serve to fully and clearly set out the associated costs in adequate detail. A life care plan also offers a critically important basis for the person and his or her family to fully appreciate the seriousness of the acquired impairments, likely complications, implications for independence and quality of life, and long-term care needs, whether for clinical or litigation purposes.[1]

For some individuals and families, a life care plan is the first and/or most comprehensive explanation of the traumatic condition and its lifelong implications. A life care plan can also be a reality check, however, placing limits on the expectations that claimants and families may develop in regard to the size and conditions of settlement. It necessarily follows that when all parties have a realistic appreciation of the nature of a condition, long-term implications, and associated realistic needs for goods and services as well as costs, early and reasonable settlements are facilitated.

Life care planners have a duty to develop a plan to assist attorneys, juries, and other health care providers in understanding the variety of special needs created by an injury and disability and how resources can be marshaled to meet those needs, including specialized care, assistive devices, medications, therapy, and environmental adaptation. In the course of preparing a plan, 1 or more of the attending physicians may be asked to work cooperatively with a life care planner in marshaling the medical evidence, identifying needs, and making lifetime prognostications. (For consistency, this article focuses on the nexus between the TBI life care planner and the physician, whether attending physician or independent expert physician. The authors recognize and acknowledge the important role of nonphysician health care professionals in life care planning, and it is appropriate for readers to infer that when physicians are referred to, it is reasonable to substitute or supplement this reference with other professionals, such as a psychologists, neuropsychologists, physiotherapists, occupational therapists, or nurses.) Alternatively, a physician who has had no prior therapeutic relationship with a patient may be retained as an independent expert by the plaintiff lawyer. Conversely, an independent expert may be retained to critically review a plaintiff's life care plan for the defense or to help prepare a second life care plan by a planner retained by the defense. In either circumstance, it is essential that physicians understand their role within the context of both the clinical development of a life care plan as well as the medicolegal setting.

Inasmuch as a life care planner has more expertise than a clinician in developing such plans, it is entirely reasonable for a planner to point out areas of omission, deficiency, and/or impracticality in clinical recommendations. The physician's role is one of expert resource and advisor to the life care planner: the physician and the planner are expected to act professionally at all times, offering impartial expertise—advocacy is never an appropriate role for an expert.

A life care plan should always be based on current standards of care and as much as possible on evidence-based practice. In a legal context, without the proper support from health care providers, a life care plan is not admissible in court. If a plan is not admissible, patients have no way of presenting vital evidence, and the result could be catastrophic: much-needed health care and ongoing support will never be considered by a jury and, thus, denied to a deserving patient.

A physician is asked by a life care planner (and later by lawyers) if the items included in the plan are reasonably necessary to manage a given injury. The physician must be guided in those opinions by conscience, professional judgment, clinical practice guidelines, and scientific evidence. The life care planner and the person with TBI depend on the physician being informed, thoughtful, deliberate, and scientifically consistent in arriving at opinions and then standing by them. A secondary consideration is that a physician will lose credibility in a courtroom for recommending an item as necessary, only to abandon that claim while under the close scrutiny or challenge of a cross-examination. The overarching goal of a physician should be to provide and recommend comprehensive, quality care for a patient. For these reasons, that goal can be achieved in litigation only by a physician who is competent, deliberate, strong, and resilient enough to withstand cross-examination.[2]

MEDICAL CONTRIBUTION TO THE TBI LIFE CARE PLAN

Life care planners come from varied backgrounds, including nursing, rehabilitation counseling, psychology, medicine, occupational, speech and physical therapy, and social work. Each life care planner presents a unique set of professional experiences and knowledge of specific disabilities. As in any field of practice, some life care planners have extensive training in life care planning methodology and knowledge specific to TBI whereas others are generalist life care planners with little training and limited knowledge of TBI. A seasoned life care planner with extensive knowledge of TBI is able to guide the discussion with the physician to ensure full and adequate consideration of all areas of future needs. Ideally, standards of practice should be adhered to as with any health care discipline or scientific methodology.[3]

For a physician working with a life care planner, it is important to understand the planner's experience in developing life care plans for the individual with TBI. Conversely, the life care planner wants to understand the physician's training and experience in TBI assessment and care. If the treating physician cannot provide the needed basis and support for the life care plan, an independent expert physician may be needed. The American Academy of Physical Medicine and Rehabilitation states that the broad medical expertise of physiatrists allows them to treat disabling conditions throughout a person's lifetime.

In working with a life care planner, a physician is asked to consider areas beyond lifelong medical care and the prevention of complications. The life care plan also addresses issues, such as therapy and durable medical equipment–related services, in the context of attempting to preserve a durable outcome for an injured party relative to productive lifestyle activities, support services, equipment needs for safety and care, therapeutic recreation, quality of life, and impact of aging. It is important for a physician working with a life care planner to understand some of the basic concepts of life care planning. Life care planners generally function under a set of guiding principles that are built around the practice of rehabilitation. Philosophic tenets that form the foundation for life care planning are outlined in Appendix 1.[4]

A well thought-out life care plan may necessitate considerable dialogue between a physician and life care planner. Physicians consulting with a life care planner must understand not only the rationale for each specific recommendation but also the relationship between each item in the plan. Life care planning is multidimensional, because each recommendation potentially affects other recommendations and elements of the plan.

The range of future care needs varies greatly depending on the severity of the TBI. Regardless of injury severity, the methodology used to examine future needs should be the same across all life care plans.[5] An advising physician must always avoid commenting on matters that fall outside that physician's scope of practice. Instead, it is reasonable and necessary to defer to other clinicians (for example, a psychiatrist defers when asked for expected orthopedic interventions or neuropsychological testing frequency and follow-up recommendations). An advising physician must be aware of all recommendations from other specialists that fall within that physician's scope of practice and must be prepared to comment, when appropriate, on causal relationship and medical necessity.

LIFE CARE PLAN DOMAINS RELEVANT TO TBI CASEWORK

When examining core components of a TBI life care plan, several critically important domains must be considered, including the following.

Home Care/Facility Care

The type and frequency of services required depend on the nature and severity of residual deficits. Services may include those from skilled nurses and unskilled care providers, life skills trainers, homemakers, and home/yard maintenance support workers. This section of the plan is typically the most expensive. Outlining the ongoing support needs of the individual with a TBI typically requires close collaboration between a physician and life care planner. Some individuals with moderate/severe TBI require ongoing home care to assist with a variety of essential services. Others with moderate/severe TBI may require long-term residential care because of the nature of their ongoing impairments, age transitions, loss of a caregiver, safety issues in the home or community, or other lifestyle changes. Such facilities or programs may provide the necessary supervisory supports, although the level of expertise provided by such programs and their per diem costs can vary significantly. It is not unusual to see several scenarios outlined within a life care plan (**Table 1** has example scenarios and their associated costs).

When analyzing family support and involvement in care, it is necessary to distinguish between the normal responsibilities of a spouse or parent and any additional forms of care or allocations of time that are related specifically to managing the consequences of the TBI. The specific type and amount of support necessary vary in

Table 1
Comparison of costs: home care assistance versus long-term support in a residential care facility

Home Care	Age/Year Initiated Through Age/Year Suspended	Hours/Shifts/Days of Care	Cost
Option 1: After brain injury rehabilitation. Home care assistance provided by a certified nursing attendant	42/2012–Life	Ages 42–50 Average of 10–12 h per d × 7 d/wk Ages 50–55 Average of 12–16 h/d × 7 d/wk Ages 55–life Average of 16–18 h/d × 7 d/wk	$16.50–$19.50/h or $180–$250/d for Live-in caregiver
Option 2: Long-term supported living in TBI residential facility	42/2012–Life	24/7 Residential living	$450–$800/d

each case and may change over time. Life care planners and clinical teams are encouraged to analyze probable risk factors and to establish viable long-term options. All cases are unique, and some may require creativity on the part of a planner and physician.

In some geographic areas, home health care services are limited and pricing is variable. In some instances, it is less expensive to hire a live-in caregiver who is paid a per diem rate as opposed to hiring a care provider paid by the hour. Depending on patient and family needs and the availability of services, there may be times when a private-hire scenario should be considered. Some families elect to independently hire private health care workers who may or may not reside in the home. Families who choose this course must be cognizant of the requirement to provide the live-in employee a private room and benefits, such as health and workers' compensation insurance coverage.

Another area often not given adequate attention is assuring optimal safety and residential and community accessibility for individuals with a brain injury within the environment in which they are cared for. Accordingly, life care planners and clinicians should keep in mind the need for adaptive equipment, such as grab bars, shower chairs, raised toilet seats, ramps, architectural modifications (including ramps), vehicular modifications for those who can drive but use wheelchairs, smoke and carbon monoxide detectors for anosmic patients, and other possible recommendations that should be considered. Other factors that should be considered in a life care plan include appropriate accommodations for caregiver and family respite if an individual with a brain injury is cared for at home. Depending on the cognitive-behavioral and physical impairment issues relevant to a case, accommodations may also need to be made for arranging special transportation (eg, a modified van), lodging, and care when on vacations.

Medication Management

Life care planners consider the medications a patient requires at the time a life care plan is developed and explore likely future use of medications as recommended by attending or expert consulting physicians. Costing for medication is typically based on retail, nondiscounted prices and should ideally include quotes for both generic and brand drugs. If a more expensive drug of the same drug class is recommended, the clinician and life care planner should both be prepared to justify why that drug and not a cheaper one from the same class, including potentially generic versions, might not be as acceptable.

Durable Medical Equipment

Many persons with TBI rely daily on durable medical equipment (DME). By reviewing past purchases of the equipment, a life care planner can understand how often an individual patient has required replacement devices in the past. If such information is not available, the planner may use Medicare guidelines for DME replacement. Marini and Harper[6] presented a study to empirically validate replacement values by surveying 101 assistive technology practitioners from across the continental United States. They analyzed data in terms of ranges, median life expectancy, and replacement parts for equipmen, and current price ranges for equipment, repairs, and maintenance.[6]

Vocational Issues

Life care planners with training and experience in developing vocational evaluations are asked to opine on an individual's ability to work. A thorough assessment may include a functional capacity evaluation, job analysis, and labor market surveys combined with consultation with other allied health professionals, including neuropsychology, psychology, occupational therapy, physical therapy, and speech therapy. For patients with TBI, the level of functional limitations affects the likelihood of return to work.[7] Other issues considered include behavioral concerns, cognitive deficits, fatigue, and deconditioning along with altered balance, vision, hearing, attention and concentration, motivation, distractibility, and bowel and bladder control as well as general mobility.

SUPPORTING RECOMMENDATIONS WITH ADEQUATE SCIENCE

A physician who is reviewing a life care plan for a patient with TBI should be aware that the plan's recommendations must always follow current evidence-based literature. Where such evidence is lacking, recommendations should be based on published guidelines or consensus opinion based on local and regional community standards of practice. Personal experience as a justification for recommendations should be avoided because it typically increases the likelihood of a legal challenge (ie, Daubert challenge) and increases the potential that testimony on said opinions or even all testimony by that expert is excluded. Drawing solely on anecdotal evidence is a dangerous practice from a medicolegal perspective: most clinicians have had limited experience with cases specific to the issue in question and, beyond that and more important, the practice is unscientific with substantial room for various forms of bias.[8]

Two levels of qualification are required of any expert testifying regarding a life care plan. First, the expert must be qualified generally in the area that he or she is opining on; and second, the expert must be qualified to substantiate—to the degree required under the particular jurisdiction's substantive law—the need for each element of care provided in the plan. Typically, the court and triers of fact look not only to the life care planner for such foundation but also to the physician who has endorsed the specific medical recommendations. (It is uncommon, but not unheard of, for a physician to obtain certification as a life care planner and thus to be able to both prepare and endorse a plan.) Therefore, the expert who is analyzing the scientific foundation of individual recommendations within a life care plan should be familiar with legal evidentiary rules and the nature of clinicolegal opinions relative to how these are interpreted and weighed by the triers of fact.

Under the US Federal Rules of Evidence, witnesses may establish their qualifications as an expert by reason of "knowledge, skill, experience, training, or education." Federal Rule 702 was written as a general grant of authority for the use of expert testimony and is, therefore, permissive in nature. Furthermore, Rule 702 stipulates that a witness who is otherwise qualified as an expert may testify in the form of an opinion or otherwise if (1) the expert scientific, technical, or other specialized knowledge will help the trier of fact to understand the evidence or to determine a fact in issue; (2) the testimony is based on sufficient facts or data; and/or (3) the testimony is the product of reliable principles and methods and the expert has reliably applied the principles and methods to the facts of the case.[9] Skills or knowledge that may be drawn on are not limited to scientific and technical areas alone but extend to all specialized knowledge. Expert testimony is generally proper in any scientific field that has reached a level of general acceptance. Most courts have at least implicitly recognized that life care planning itself has reached such a degree of general acceptance as to be the proper subject of expert testimony. Thus, expert testimony is generally permitted in conjunction with a life care plan.

A lack of adequate factual foundation likely results in an expert's testimony stricken as based on speculation.[10] Such an issue may arise if, for example, a life care planner intends to testify regarding the cost of certain treatment, but no medical evidence has been proffered to indicate that such treatment is reasonable, necessary, or caused by the relevant accident or mishap (eg, substandard care). Such foundation objections likely are considered in cases where objections to a life care planner's qualifications have been overruled (the general legal defense principle is to attack the legitimacy of both the message and the messenger). The speculative nature of a life care plan can also preclude its admissibility if the plan involves new or experimental treatments or novel theories of causation.[11]

All opinions need to be stated with a degree of probability. Occasionally, the term, *degree of certainty*, is used by lawyers and judges; however, case law does not differentiate degree of certainty from degree of probability relative to a difference in statistical thresholds for the likelihood of the occurrence discussed. Both terms are used to indicate that an event is more likely than not to occur. More specifically, when stating something with a degree of medical probability, it simply means that the chance of the occurrence of that condition is greater than 50%. To make such statements, adequate evidence is needed. Unfortunately, many opinions of this nature are provided without adequate scientific foundation.

Individuals with a brain injury who are suing for damages (ie, claimants) have the burden of establishing that the pertinent admissibility requirements are met by a preponderance of evidence. The specific criteria for admitting scientific expert testimony explicated by Daubert are (1) whether an expert's technique or theory can be or has been tested—that is, whether the expert's theory can be challenged or refuted in some objective sense or whether it is simply a subjective conclusion that cannot reasonably be refuted or assessed for reliability; (2) whether the technique or theory has been subject to peer review and publication; (3) the known or potential rate of error of the technique or theory when applied; (4) the existence and maintenance of standards and controls; and, (5) the degree to which the technique or theory has been generally accepted in the scientific community.[12] Not all of the specific Daubert factors can apply to every type of expert testimony. The Daubert challenge strategy is increasingly used to challenge both life care planning and medical professional testimony in brain injury cases. When an expert purports to apply principles and methods in accordance with professional standards, yet reaches a conclusion that other experts in the field would not reach, the trial court may reasonably conclude that the principles and methods have not been faithfully applied. In such cases, any step that renders the analysis unreliable also render the expert's testimony inadmissible. This is true whether the step completely changes the reliable methodology or merely misapplies that methodology.

Scientific evidence is relevant when there is a valid scientific connection to the pertinent inquiry as a precondition to admissibility. It is of utmost importance to point out that ethically, medicolegally, and morally, if a clinician or life care planner is to testify regarding a claimant who is alive, then that individual has an obligation to directly examine the party involved in the litigation and not base testimony solely on review of the medical records. Peer reviews should be used internally by the requesting party, and such reviews should not be substituted for direct examination and/or serve as a basis for testimony. One exception to this rule is in death cases; however, in such situations, a life care plan generally is irrelevant, although there are always exceptions. In such death cases, issues of lost wages, loss of consortium (loss of consortium is considered a valid claim in the United States but is not recognized by Canadian courts), pain, and suffering as well as other issues might be relevant from a forensic and clinicolegal standpoint.

Ideally, unless a life care plan is authored by an appropriately qualified physician, which is rarely the case, the plan must faithfully cite the medical sources for all specific medical recommendations. In addition, the overall plan should be endorsed by a physician to provide additional bolstering to the life care planner's opinions on medical necessity and the causal relationship with the litigated issues. When a life care planner can also justify recommendations with scientific publications that are methodologically sound or publications that summarize such data, such as reference textbooks, then the opinions are further supported and that much more incontrovertible.

COMMON FAUX PAS IN TBI LIFE CARE PLAN CASEWORK
Probability and Timeframe Issues

The authors of this article have seen several common errors in life care plans over their respective careers, which cumulatively are nearly 100 years of practice. One common but major error is the failure to make a clear differentiation between possibility and probability when considering the risk of a future event. It is critical for experts to exercise caution in identifying each event that occurs with a degree of medical probability, as opposed to those for which there is merely an increased risk (possibility), because triers of fact consider compensable only those complications that are probable. Possible complications may be listed in the plan for the sake of completeness, but these are not considered compensable. A related concern is an unwarranted endorsement of a possible complication or time frame for neurologic change after a TBI as probable, despite the absence of scientific data to support such a claim.

Some examples of issues that may arise in a life care plan that demonstrate the application of bad science can be found in the following statements:

- The patient will likely remain at risk for developing communicating hydrocephalus beyond the first year posttrauma.
- Because this patient has sustained a severe TBI, it remains likely that he or she will develop a posttraumatic seizure disorder beyond 5 years postinjury.
- It is likely that this patient will develop dementia as a result of his or her mild brain injury.
- It is likely that the patient will develop heterotopic ossification that is functionally limiting even beyond the first year postinjury.
- The patient has been in a minimally conscious state for 3 years. Because it is likely that the patient will eventually recover from this state, the life care plan must factor in that extensive neurorehabilitation services will be required for the rest of the patient's life span.
- The patient has sustained a severe brain injury and is in a vegetative or minimally conscious state. The life care plan provisions are based on the understanding that the median survival time or life expectancy will not be affected and instead are the same as in the general, non–brain-injured population.[13]

Laboratory Studies

Another often-challenged area of life care plan testimony deals with the scientific basis for recommendations for laboratory work. Concerns include whether laboratory work related to the injury-related medications is necessary and, if it is necessary, whether the frequency for testing is reasonable. Generally, there are published standards for laboratory monitoring of particular drugs, but it may surprise many to learn of the lack of solid evidence-based medicine for a specific frequency of performing many commonly used laboratory studies for various medications. An example is the monitoring of antiepileptic drugs for hepatotoxic and hematologic side effects. Another concern is inappropriate inclusion in a life care plan of laboratory testing that would have been done anyway as part of general health care or because of noncompensable medication treatment.

Medication Management

Often, life care plans include medications recommended for long-term use despite a lack of scientific data supporting long-term use in such a context. Additionally, it is difficult if not impossible to make predictions, particularly early after injury, about how long a given patient may need to be on a particular medication. There are some exceptions, such as patients whose duration and frequency of seizures permit the conclusion that it is probable that lifetime treatment with an antiepileptic medication will be necessary. Drug classes that may be controversial as to their need for long-term management include psychotropic medications, such as neuroleptics and antidepressants as well as other mood stabilizers, including certain antiepileptic drugs and lithium.

Another frequent life care planning issue in litigation over TBI cases is whether a recommended medication is clinically warranted and efficacious for treating a particular claimed impairment. Frequently, a life care plan lists 1 or more medications currently prescribed to a particular patient with brain injury that have not, at least on chart review, been shown to make a substantive difference in that person's functional abilities and/or clearly substantiated relative to its clinical purpose. It is important for life care planners to challenge physicians as to the need for each prescribed medication and determine if adequate evidence of a positive clinical response justifies its inclusion in the life care plan.

Last, medications are often used off-label in TBI care and for non–FDA-approved indications. Physicians, as well as life care planners, need to be prepared to justify the medical necessity of using off-label medications to the triers of fact. In such circumstances, testifying experts likely need to rely on practice trends in the field or published consensus guidelines that may not have a substantive evidence-based foundation.

Care Needs

The amount of supervision and/or professional care an individual with TBI requires, based on claimed functional level, may generate the most debate of all areas in a life care plan. A person's cognitive, behavioral, and physical limitations must be considered in the context of his or her living environment, the validity and reliability of historical records, injury data, patient/claimant performance on examinations (whether clinical or in the context of independent evaluations), naturalistic observations, and corroboratory reports when making probabilistic determinations about need for future care. Often, the most debated topic is predicting how patients will function in the community, assuming this is where they will be living or where they are living. Sometimes, arguments center on the disparity between functional difficulties observed in the community versus the relatively better performance seen on tests, such as neuropsychological examinations. Issues of ecological validity, however, must be understood by all involved parties and the facts associated with same appreciated; that is, sometimes people perform better on structured neuropsychological examinations administered in quiet, nondistracting environments but may function poorly when living in the real world, where they require more executive function skills.

Life care plans often stipulate substantive to excessive recommendations for the types of professional care that is necessary. These may involve both frequency and duration for therapeutic services as well as multidisciplinary medical services, such as physiatry, neurology, neurosurgery, psychiatry, and so forth. Ideally, life care planners should identify necessary services and establish frequencies and then try to consolidate medical care to make it as convergent as possible, given the problems associated with divergent care.

One such area of concern involves recommendations made for frequent therapeutic services spanning excessively long periods of time despite a lack of indication of clinical efficacy for a patient or any evidence-based medicine to support the practice. This is of particular concern in life care plans for patients who have incurred single, concussive brain injuries.

For more severely disabled patients, controversies often abound about the type of direct care staffing necessary, ranging from uncertified/unskilled "hires off the street" to licensed staff, including certified nursing assistants, licensed practical nurses, and registered nurses. There are no good research studies analyzing and recommending the types of care for particular types of patients; typically, the life care planner needs to defer to the local nursing standards with regard to the nature of the care rendered. For example, patients who require tracheostomy care, *percutaneous endoscopic gastrostomy* care, or administration of medications via *percutaneous endoscopic gastrostomy* need higher levels of certified nursing personnel support than patients who have none of those needs. These recommendations must be critically analyzed not only in regard to the type of person providing care but also the frequency and duration for which such individuals need to be present to provide such care.

Defense attorneys, not infrequently, try to suggest that a family should assume caretaker roles for their loved ones with more catastrophic brain injury. Family members and significant others should, generally, not take on the dual roles of loved ones and caretakers. Every attempt should be made to optimally preserve the normal relationship of the persons with brain injury with their significant others, including avoiding the pitfall of making loved ones caretakers.

Adequate Follow-Up

The biggest disservice the legal process can do to an injured party with a TBI is to underestimate and undervalue the type of lifelong medical care that may be necessary to support that individual. Less sophisticated or insufficiently informed clinicians and/or life care planners may be remiss in including within the TBI life care plan both appropriate medical and rehabilitative treatment and reasonable follow-up. The life care plan must adequately address medication, laboratory, and DME costs as well as repair and replacement costs, likely future surgeries (eg, shunt replacement), life expectancy, needs for maintenance therapy, and medical follow-up costs, among other issues.

CAVEATS FOR REVIEWING TBI LIFE CARE PLANS

Not uncommonly, independent expert clinicians may be asked to review a life care plan. The request may originate with a life care planner, particularly during the process of preparation, when unusual or complex issues require clarification or further exploration that cannot be obtained from busy attending clinicians. Some life care planners work as a team with independent specialists who can expedite data assembly or otherwise facilitate the development of a plan. The request may instead originate with legal counsel (plaintiff or defense), looking for either an independent endorsement of a life care plan they have commissioned or an independent review of a life care plan that has been commissioned by the opposing lawyer.

When a physician is asked to evaluate a life care plan, a systematic top-down approach is typically advisable. This begins by fully reviewing a plan's overview of the history, injuries, and impairments, to determine if the planner has adequately grasped the issues, and then goes on to determine if the proposed services follow logically, are supported by citations from the attending caregivers, and are warranted by scientific evidence.

If this review finds critical shortcomings, the expert should not hesitate to indicate the sources of concern to the referring planner or lawyer. If critical errors are found, an expert should not hesitate to refuse to endorse the components that are of concern or even the entire plan if necessary. In fairness, when retained by the same counsel who commissioned the life care plan, the expert might wish to consider offering to assist the planner with remediation of the critical errors, leading to a life care plan the expert can endorse.

Some of the questions that physician reviewers should ask themselves when assessing the quality of a life care plan on a patient or claimant with a TBI include, but are not necessarily limited to, the following:

1. Does the planner demonstrate a good grasp of the medical issues in question?
2. What were the planner's sources of information?
   a. Does it seem that the planner has consulted with an appropriate range of key caregivers?
   b. Has each consultation been in adequate depth?
   c. Has the planner adequately set out the information actually provided and relied on, and do the recommendations of the clinicians correspond closely with what the plan contains?
   d. Is the planner relying on an insufficient set of advising clinicians?
   e. As a corollary, it is appropriate to ask whether the planner has relied on problematically unscientific guidance from any of these sources or on sources whose opinions either fall outside their scope of practice or are unrepresentative of common practices.
3. Is the detail about the claimant sufficient and reliable, including education, work background, domestic situation, and family?
4. Is the list of impairments and related needs comprehensive and realistic?
5. Does the list of proposed goods and services flow logically from the list of impairments and needs?
6. Is the planner offering any generic, off-the-shelf information without appropriate clinical confirmation?

Some triers of fact are particularly astute at using such considerations and rejecting unfounded provisions; others may not be particularly critical and instead require education from expert critiques. A flawed life care plan can be effectively challenged in its entirety, or at least in regards to its weaker elements, when opposing counsel is sophisticated and/or the defense experts are knowledgeable in their fields of expertise. In a worst-case scenario, such challenges can lead to the exclusion of the plan and/or an expert's testimony.

In general, when reviewing a life care plan, experts should avoid addressing services that they have limited knowledge about, as is the case for any area outside their domain of expertise. If an expert has previously been disqualified in a TBI case because of a Daubert challenge, this may reduce both credibility in the clinicolegal arena and ability to be accepted as an expert in other cases.

It is reasonable for clinicians to consider whether the services that do fall within their area of expertise seem causally relatable to the injury or event in question, are medically necessary, and are based on realistic market values obtained by canvassing multiple sources for the region in which a patient or claimant lives. An expert may find that some goods or services are exceptionally unusual within the context of a claimant's diagnosis or are to be provided at frequencies and durations that fall well outside common practices or likely benefit.

Typically, a review of the actual costs is not within the purview of a clinician, unless the clinician has special familiarity or expertise in this area. Sometimes an expert may find that although each component of a plan seems reasonable when considered in isolation, overall the plan provisions are excessive in the time and effort required of the patient each day, leading to fatigue, reduced lifestyle independence, or increased dependency on therapists.

Some impairments require constant or frequent supply of goods or services; other impairments may have infrequent care needs, which are nevertheless serious when present. As a result, a plan should make clear whether the frequency of provision of a good or service is calendar driven or needs driven. For example, if a patient's obesity is an obstacle to mobility, a patient may be deemed as needing a long-term weight management program with nutritional counseling. It is reasonable for the plan to initially fund a regular weekly (ie, calendar driven) visit with a nutritionist, to review diet, set up a meal plan, discuss healthy food habits, and so forth. If a claimant shows good retention of what is taught by the nutritionist, then over the long term nutritionist visits can be shifted to a need-driven schedule, with funding made available for occasional appointments in association with unusual needs (such as onset of a medical complication, surgery, and so forth) or a wish for comprehensive review to address backsliding or effects of aging. In contrast, specialized dental surveillance and care (such as managing gum hyperplasia associated with long-term Dilantin use) is typically entirely calendar driven for life.

Overassessing or overservicing impairments is a common problem in life care plans. After a moderate TBI, neuropsychological testing at 6 months and again at 2 years typically establishes the nature of the impairments and the extent of recovery during the first 2 years, leading to an accurate appreciation of persisting neurocognitive sequelae and a reasonable extrapolation of long-term needs. A life care plan that calls for repeat neuropsychological testing every 2 years for life, as advised by an attending neurologist but without justification for same, likely is effectively challenged in court.

Sometimes a diagnosis remains unclear or unverified years after onset. As an example, a clinician is asked to review a life care plan in which the plaintiff had been diagnosed by a family doctor with a moderately severe TBI and was claiming pronounced impairment and disablement. The diagnosis and claims led the planner to propose extensive TBI-oriented support services and substantial cost allowances. The reviewing expert, however, finds that the evidence within the medical records is most consistent with a diagnosis of not greater than uncomplicated concussion and that substantial to complete recovery should have taken place. The diagnosis was never confirmed by any qualified specialist, such as a neurologist or physiatrist, and the claimed impairments and the needs outlined in the life care plan were well out of line with any reasonable sequelae. In this case, a critical review of the life care plan might benefit from a contingency-based, multimodal approach based on the consideration that the trier of fact might make 1 of 3 findings:

1. There was either no TBI or at most transient sequelae because of a concussion, with no possibility of any persistent, functionally significant sequelae,
2. There was a TBI and although sequelae were possible, they would not be functionally significant.
3. There was a sufficient TBI for functionally significant sequelae to be likely.

By addressing all 3 contingencies, a clinical review is valid and useful, notwithstanding which finding is eventually made. Concerning the first contingency, the reviewer merely indicates that because the evidence is consistent with the inference that either there had been no TBI, or at least there was no possibility of neurologic sequelae, the entire life care plan should be considered to have no neurologic basis. As for the second contingency, if it were assumed that at worst the claimant had a concussion with modest sequelae, then only certain specific proposals could be considered reasonable within the context of a mild TBI. Here, the report goes on to identify and review these within this section. In the third contingency, the report posits that if it is assumed that the claim in its entirety was credible, then a comprehensive review of necessity and reasonableness of the plan in its entirety is applicable, and the report provides that analysis with respect to the third contingency.

Sometimes a reviewing physician finds that the predicate assumptions of diagnosis and impairment severity on which a life care plan is based are potentially invalid. The relevance of the written critique to the parties and to the court depends on whether the triers of fact endorse the assumptions in whole or in part. One approach to preparing the critique is to take a contingency-based approach, by addressing each provision from the perspective of each of several diagnostic possibilities.

For example, a defense lawyer requests a critique of a life care plan for a woman diagnosed by her general practitioner as having a moderately severe TBI but which has not been confirmed by any specialist. She is claiming pronounced disablement, and the planner retained by the plaintiff lawyer has proposed extensive TBI-oriented support services at substantial cost. The reviewing physician finds that the evidence suggests that the original injury was at most a mild concussion with transient neurologic symptoms and a large apparent psychological overlay with potential for symptom magnification. Accordingly, aside from treatment of possible persistent postconcussion symptoms, nothing in the extensive life care plan is reasonable. The defense lawyer advises, however, that because trials are unpredictable and a trier of fact might find that a moderately severe TBI had occurred, a contingency-based analysis by the expert would be most helpful. The physician prepares the critique accordingly, first commenting on the reasonableness of the life care plan as a whole and then on each provision incrementally. Thus, the critique would set out, in overview fashion, the following facts:

1. The evidence strongly indicates that there was either no TBI or at most a mild concussion with transient sequelae from which full recovery is the most likely outcome. If that is so, then the life care plan, in its entirety, is completely inapplicable to the case in question.
2. It is acknowledged that a small percentage of patients after mild TBI or concussion may have persistent postconcussive symptoms. If that is the eventual finding in the case, then the only relevant sections of the life care plan are those that deal with investigating and/or managing symptoms of headache and dizziness, which are most likely related at this time to the concussion sustained in the accident in question and/or to associated injury involving the head or neck. The balance of the life care plan is inapplicable to the case in question.
3. To accommodate the possibility of an eventual finding of a more serious TBI, however, each provision of the life care plan is reviewed for reasonableness, strictly on the basis of, at most, a mild–moderate TBI.

Appendix 2 provides an example of a complete, critical medical review of a life care plan.

SUMMARY

Life care plans for persons with TBI require a thorough comprehension of the scope of problems that are associated with this condition. That scope is particularly broad, because it may involve motor deficits, cognitive and communication impairments, neuropsychiatric problems, fatigue, central pain, and other aspects. Appropriate life care planning development relies heavily on a thoroughly detailed approach to encompassing the multidimensionality of the myriad issues facing persons with TBI-related impairments and associated handicaps. The need for specialist physician input in the development of life care plans is a crucial piece to assuring a solid scientific foundation for justification of the costs associated with same as well as the life care plan's contents. Life care planners and physician specialists should be intimately familiar with both their clinical and medicolegal roles and obligations, ethically, medically, and morally.

A comprehensive understanding of the neuromedical and neurorehabilitative needs of this patient population is of utmost importance in serving as a foundation for developing comprehensive and accurate TBI life care plans. When in doubt regarding the science, appropriate resources should be consulted, including peer-reviewed literature and/or core reference textbooks in the field.[14,15]

REFERENCES

1. Kreuscher WC. Rational life care planning. J Life Care Plan 2010;9(1):3–14.
2. Zasler ND. A physiatric perspective on life care planning. NARPS Journal 1994; 9(2&3):57–61.
3. Reavis N, Preston K, Weed R. International Academy of Life Care Planners (IALCP)—Standards of Practice. Available at: www.rehabpro.org/sections/ialcp/focus/standards/IALCP%20-%20Standards%20of%20Practice.pdf. Accessed September 8, 2012.
4. Deutsch PM, Allison L, Reid C. An introduction to life care planning: history, tenets, methodologies, and principles. Chapter 5. In: Deutsch PM, Sawyer HW, editors. A guide to rehabilitation. White Plains (NY): AHAB Press; 2003. p. 5-1–5-61.
5. Weed RO, Berens DE. Life care planning after traumatic brain injury: clinical and forensic issues. In: Zasler N, Katz D, Zafonte R, et al, editors. Brain injury medicine: principles and practice. New York: Demos Medical Publishing; 2013. p. 1437–54.
6. Marini I, Harper D. Empirical validation of medical equipment replacement values in life care plans. J Life Care Plan 2010;4(4):173–82.
7. Wehman P, Kregel J, Sherron P, et al. Critical factors associated with successful supported employment placement of patients with severe traumatic brain injury. Brain Inj 1993;7(1):31–44.
8. Fagel BG. Proving and obtaining reasonable damages in medical malpractice cases. Forum Magazine 2011;41(3):20–2.
9. Cornell University Law School. Federal Rules of Evidence: Rule 702. Testimony By Expert Witnesses. Legal Information Institute. Available at: www.law.cornell.edu/rules/fre/rule_702. Accessed August 5, 2012.
10. Patterson RM. An irreverent look at life care planners. J Life Care Plan 2010;9(1):19–40.
11. Washington AD. Attacking the life care plan—a common sense approach. Products, General Liability and Consumer Law Committee Newsletter Spring 2010;4–6.

12. Wikipedia. Daubert standard. Available at: http://en.wikipedia.org/wiki/Daubert_standard. Accessed August 14, 2012.
13. Zasler ND. Long-term survival after severe TBI: clinical and forensic aspects. Prog Brain Res 2009;177:111–24.
14. Silver JM, McAllister TW, Yudofsky SC, editors. Textbook of traumatic brain injury. 2nd edition. Washington, DC: American Psychiatric Publishing; 2011.
15. Zasler ND, Katz DI, Zafonte R, editors. Brain injury medicine: principles and practice. 2nd edition. New York: Demos Medical Publishers; 2013.
16. Thomas RL, Kitchen J. Private hire: the real costs. Inside Life Care Planning 1996; 1(3):3–4.

APPENDIX 1: THE BASIC TENETS OF LIFE CARE PLANNING

1. *First and foremost, life care planners are rehabilitation professionals and educators.* The role of a life care planner is that of educator, not advocate. When developing a plan, a planner must maintain objectivity and base recommendations on research literature, the opinions of consulting team members (physicians, therapists, and so forth), and patient-specific data. The responsibility of the life care planners is to set forth attainable rehabilitation goals and to ensure that all parties involved in the process understand why specific items are included, how and when services should be provided, and how a plan is best implemented.

2. *All plan recommendations should clearly relate to patient-specific evaluation data.* It is essential that each recommendation is carefully linked to the data collected in the clinical interview and history taken with patients and families as well as in the review of all medical/health-related professional records. The basis for each item citation should be clear to others who review the life care plan; no one should be left to wonder why specific recommendations were made.

3. *Assume the probability of success of recommendations.* It is inappropriate to make recommendations in a plan, then proceed as though those recommendations are not going to be successful. If the recommendations are worthy of inclusion, it is appropriate to assume the probability of their success. The plan should be built on successful outcomes.

4. *Life care plans are designed to answer questions, not raise them.* A life care plan should be self-explanatory. If it is not, revisions should be made so all can understand it easily. A format should be developed that uses a natural writing style but is also reader friendly. Use explanations in the comment box and footnote sections wherever necessary. Have a team member review the plan and objectively comment on the readability of the document. This is critical when a plan is referred to within a general case management setting. It improves communications and reduces the time spent in deposition if a plan is scrutinized within a forensics setting. Clarity of communication with patients, families, and interested third parties is critical so that recommendations are not misinterpreted or misapplied.

5. *Life care plans specify provisions throughout life expectancy and cannot depend on any one individual, service, or supplier to fulfill plan recommendations.* Always use at least 3 sources for the major cost items in the plan. Do not use negotiated rates because there is no guarantee that the cost remains constant if a business or supplier should change hands. Life care planners should not habitually seek discounted rates for repeat referrals. Costs should reflect real values of goods and services found within a patient's local market. Also, eliminate outliers from the market analysis so that unrealistically low or high rates do not misrepresent the actual cost of an item.

6. *Recommendations must consider disability, individual, family, and regional factors.* Make sure the services recommended are available in a patient's geographic location. If they are not, include transportation expenses or develop a program using area resources. For example, if the patient lives in a rural setting with few paved sidewalks, the wheelchair recommended should be durable within that environment. Life care plans are never generic: always consider individual variables that make a plan a custom fit to a patient and family.

7. *Attend to details.* A clearly written, well-documented life care plan and a professional image are significant steps toward credibility. Strive to maintain professionalism and to produce a professional product. Carefully proof all work for careless spelling, mathematical, grammatical, and terminological errors. Evaluate the narrative report, life care plan, and all correspondence for internal consistency and ensure that the recommendations progress in a logical sequence. The plan is a tool of communication, not confusion: remember that the referral source, patient, and family are not likely to be familiar with the terminology, acronyms, medical codes, abbreviations, and nomenclature taken for granted by a planner.

8. *Recommendations are proactive, not reactive.* Life care plans should be developed and implemented to prevent the frequency of occurrence, severity, and duration of complications. The recommendations must be clearly related to evaluation data identifying specific individual needs and must be expected to benefit the individual. If an individual is not expected to benefit from a given service or piece of equipment, then that recommendation should not be made. If a recommendation is expected to benefit an individual, however, the expected benefit should be considered in developing the rest of the plan. For example, if an individual with paraplegia but no history of decubiti is provided appropriate wheelchair cushioning and training regarding pressure release, skin inspection, and other methods to prevent the development of decubiti, that individual's life care plan should not include provisions for 4 surgeries per year to treat decubiti. The assumption is that the best care and recommendations will work and such complications will not occur because of preventive intervention. Assuming otherwise suggests that complications can be accurately predicted despite the lack of a statistical basis for that assumption and furthermore fails to consider the impact such an assumption has on ongoing complications that may affect life expectancy.

9. *Recognize the benefits of maximizing patient potential.* In addition to individual quality-of-life benefits, financial benefits may result from maximizing rehabilitation outcomes through the provision of timely and appropriate services. Consider the following example. Imagine the costs over a lifetime for 2 different 24-year-old individuals, both with C5-C6 spinal cord injuries. One person can turn himself at night or can tolerate 6 hours without being turned; the other cannot. The difference in expected lifetime costs reduced to present value for these 2 individuals is more than $2 million. This difference is based on patients' functional limitations and the degree to which their levels of independence affect staffing requirements for support care.

10. *Life care planning is multidimensional.* Life care planning is multidimensional, because each recommendation potentially affects other recommendations and elements of the plan. Driven by a specific functional limitation or impairment, all items cited within a plan affect other recommendations both directly and indirectly. For example, multiple disabilities and multiple service providers might dictate similar recommendations, resulting in service overlaps or duplications. Consider the effects of a change from intermittent catheterization every 4 to 6 hours to a suprapubic catheterization program for a C5 tetraplegic who is not

independent in self-catheterization. With intermittent catheterization, a patient requires a licensed practical nurse to perform the procedure. Visiting nurses are impractical because the program would require 4 to 5 visits every 24 hours, plus the cost of visiting nurses precludes this form of care from being a realistic, fiscally responsible option. Two 12-hour shifts or three 8-hour shifts of skilled nursing care are necessary. If a change to a suprapubic catheter is required, however, this skilled nursing care need can be met with nursing visits for the patient's bowel program every other day, at which time a nurse can also flush the suprapubic tube. This nursing arrangement can also accommodate a once-per-month suprapubic tube change.

11. *Consider the entire cost of each recommendation.* Life care plan developers as well as case managers implementing these plans need to consider all costs associated with a given service option or piece of equipment. For equipment, the overall cost must take into account the cost of maintenance and the necessary frequency of replacement. This is particularly true when calculating the cumulative cost of assistive technology and equipment that makes use of consumable supplies. Thomas and Kitchen[16] compared the costs of hiring a personal care attendant through an agency versus privately hiring one. When the total costs (including employer Social Security and Medicare matches, state unemployment taxes, fringe benefits, payroll expenses, background checks, appropriate supervision, and so forth) of a private hire are considered, the appeal of hiring through an agency increases. In addition to the modifications within the home care element of the plan, changes would also be required in supplies, routine, invasive medical care, and possibly medication.

12. *The costs provided in a life care plan do not include 2 important categories: potential complications and future technology.* The costs associated with these areas cannot be predicted accurately. The degree to which complications are experienced or future technology developed to meet a given individual's needs cannot be known; therefore, these costs are not included in the final cost analysis of life care plans. It is important, however, for life care planners and case managers to inform decision makers of the potential for development of complications as well as invention of future technology, both of which could have an impact even though they have not been included in the life care plan projections. Within the narrative report or the life care plan, the planners should clearly state that the issues of complications and technological advancement were not ignored but rather that no valid method of calculating the costs and needs associated with either area exists. Life care planners must be certain to educate others and indicate that recommendations are based on what has been determined to occur within reasonable rehabilitation probability. Events that lie beyond the realm of reasonable rehabilitation probability simply cannot be evaluated accurately.

13. *Consider the psychological effects of the injury or disability.* Psychological factors have a significant impact on the quality of life for individuals with catastrophic injuries. Making an individual a part of the decision-making team early in the process, no matter his or her level of participation, is critical to the success of plan implementation. Having choices and exercising control over one's environment are especially important for individuals with catastrophic injuries that interfere with mobility and physical function. For example, installation of an environmental control unit is a psychological intervention, an aid for independent functioning, and a safety precaution. If a tetraplegic individual has a personal care attendant available to turn the channels on a television or to dial a telephone, for example, a naïve individual might question the need for a voice-activated system to operate

those items. The psychological importance of restoring as much choice and independent control over one's environment as possible, however, should not be underestimated. Psychological interventions should take into consideration the current demonstrated needs of an individual and his or her family as well as future adjustments expected over the life span. For an adult who is injured, adjustments are expected during critical life phases, such as marriage, beginning a family, and retirement. For children with disabilities, appropriate short-term psychological goals should be established for different developmental stages.

14. *Disability interacts with age to produce additional concerns.* Psychological aspects vary with age, as do physical aspects of function. When disability interacts with the aging process, specific body parts are known to wear out faster than they do for individuals without a disability.

APPENDIX 2: A CRITICAL PHYSICIAN REVIEW OF A LIFE CARE PLAN

The following are extracts of a critical physician review of a life care plan for a patient who, notwithstanding a highly questionable history (ie, it is doubtful that any brain injury occurred as a result of her accident), has made claims of profound posttraumatic neurologic impairment and disability. The plaintiff planner has matched these claims with what can most charitably be described as a sympathetic and generous, off-the-shelf major brain injury life care plan.

1. The life care planner states that the basis of her life care plan is her understanding that Ms X sustained a moderately severe TBI and, in consequence, is unable to work, care for her family or household, or perform many aspects of instrumental or even personal activities of daily living, instead requiring substantial housekeeping and attendant care.

2. In reviewing her file, however, the physician does not find the requisite medical basis for the claimed injury and impairments. In regard to the severity of the claimed TBI, Ms X's neurologist diagnosed only a mild TBI. Her own neuropsychologist noted that test results were highly variable 1-year postonset, and she concluded that the claimant may have had a mild to moderate head injury, not a moderately severe injury. A psychiatrist's report concludes that the presentation is more in keeping with a pseudodementia of depression. Moreover, although Ms X reported to many physicians that she had lost consciousness in the accident, the ambulance attendant record clearly states, "patient knocked to ground by turning school bus, no loss of consciousness," which is inconsistent with an injury more serious than a mild TBI. The attending emergency department orthopedist commented, "I suspect she just had an elbow and cervical strain."

3. Therefore, it is clear that at most Ms X might have sustained a concussion (ie, a mild TBI) without an associated loss of consciousness. Current understanding of mild TBI is that most people recover completely, but a subset may have persistent postconcussive symptoms. Although a persistent postconcussive symptoms might justify some modest longer-term services that could be put into a life care plan, the conceivable sequelae in no way account for the level of dependency claimed. Although the physician acknowledges that the neuropsychologist diagnosed a mild–moderate TBI, it is also relevant that within the literature there is some doubt as to whether neuropsychological testing has a discrimination rate better than 50:50 (random) for mild (as opposed to moderate or worse) TBI.

4. Although the physician's review of the plan leads to the conclusion that the claimant either did not sustain any injury or is at most suffering from a mild TBI, the physician reviews the necessity and reasonableness of the various provisions

of this life care plan with reference to both injury possibilities: a mild TBI or mild–moderate TBI.

5. Medications—The life care plan proposes celecoxib, acetaminophen, and duloxetine. Analgesia may help with postconcussive headaches, and depression can be a postconcussive problem. Both classes of drugs are used to treat both mild TBI and mild–moderate TBI. Neither class of drugs is necessary, however, from an accident perspective, if the concussion has fully resolved.

6. Topicals—Lakota cream and efficascent oil are proposed for widespread benign chronic pain. According to the literature, neither topical preparation has any known efficacy and may be only placebos. Moreover, the chronic pain is said to be diffuse, whereas the initial elbow and neck strains have resolved and are not the foci of local pain. Consequently, the physician does not regard these as necessary or reasonable and certainly neither is indicated for mild TBI or mild–moderate TBI. The source of prescription for these topicals is not cited by the planner and seems instead an instance of either self-medication or else reflecting the planner's own recommendations, neither of which is acceptable for a life care plan.

7. Scheduler—An iPad and monthly contract with lifetime renewals are proposed. No caregiver is identified as source for the recommendation and no justification is given for an iPad. The physician questions why an iPad, specifically, has been designated as helpful for scheduling. Many other electronic and paper solutions are available for scheduling; thus, the proposal is incomplete, poorly justified, and/or not necessary.

8. Assistive devices—The life care planner proposes a cane, high-back support, leg massager, heat gel pack, orthopedic mattress (cost differential only), and soap dispensers. The planner cites a physiotherapist's report for the recommendations. The physician reviews this report and the medical reports and it is clear that the claimant did not sustain serious physical injury and has no neurologic finding of imbalance. Her cervical strain has healed. In reviewing the physiotherapist report, there is no connection between any findings set out in that report and the recommendations, which instead seem based on vague diagnostic assumptions and on symptom self-report. None of these is necessary based on the facts of the case even if she had a mild TBI or mild–moderate TBI. None is necessary after minor soft tissue strains or particularly efficacious for treating chronic pain.

9. Urologic—A lifetime supply of panty liners is proposed. The universally acknowledged sequelae of persistent impairments from mild TBI do not include incontinence. It is atypical for mild–moderate TBI, but, in any event, no medical diagnosis of posttraumatic incontinence is documented anywhere in the file. Urinary incontinence has many idiopathic etiologies, and incontinence is surprisingly prevalent within the general population. Treatments, such as Kegel exercises, should be tried before consigning a person to a lifetime of requiring panty liners. The physician concludes that the proposal is not necessary or reasonable for Ms X.

10. Bath chair and stationary bike—These recommendations were made by Ms X's physiotherapist. A bath chair is helpful with orthopedic chronic pain but unnecessary in regard to any conceivable neurologic sequelae in this case. Although a stationary bike might offer fitness and weight control, it is well known that compliance with home exercise programs and equipment is low. Moreover, socialization, education, and supervision as well as regular scheduling have important benefits for pain, emotional health, and fitness, so the physician instead supports a health club membership. Many patients with mild–moderate TBI benefit from such

programs because they can improve fitness, balance, and weight, among other benefits.

11. Cell phone plan—Cell phones can be useful for people with moderate to severe TBI that experience confusion and problems of disorientation or wandering. Even if Ms X had sustained a mild–moderate TBI, however, she has never shown confusion or wandering. A cell phone, therefore, is not indicated in this case. Moreover, cell phones have become ubiquitous, and provision of one is not medically justifiable in this case.

12. Therapies—The plan proposes that Ms X receive sufficient funds for occupational therapy and a rehabilitative support worker for annual services after a more intensive initial program. It is 5 years since the accident. Ms X has been regularly receiving occupational therapy services but has not benefited to date. The physician concludes that that the current intense program does not demonstrate any potential for benefit. Neither provision is reasonable if she had had a mild TBI. Even if her TBI was mild–moderate, the physician can find no evidence of potential benefit at this late date.

13. Counseling—The proposal for lifetime counseling services originated with the social worker who has been counseling her twice per week for the past 4 years. The planner has not cited either the attending neuropsychologist or the psychiatrist, who has been periodically consulted for depression management. Counseling to date has had no discernible benefit. Lifetime counseling is not appropriate for either mild TBI or mild–moderate TBI; thus, the physician concludes that this proposal is not reasonable.

14. Vision therapy—The physician can find no clinical source for this proposal. Ms X saw an ophthalmologist 2 years after the accident, complaining of headaches, photosensitivity, and dry eyes. The examination found that poor fixation had confounded testing and suggested the presence of functional overlay in an otherwise normal eye examination. The physician concludes that this proposal is not medically supported and is not reasonable. Travel to vision therapy is also not reasonable.

15. Case management—Case management is not reasonable for typical persons with mild TBI and is not indicated in this particular case; however, it is justifiable for a person with mild–moderate TBI, if impairment of judgment or other cognitive functions was present and/or there were numerous complex issues that required follow-up and coordination. Because this is not the case, however, the physician does not support the need for case management.

16. Housing assessment—The plan proposes that living in a bungalow would be easier and safer for Ms X than living in her current 4-story home. The proposal did not originate with any caregiver. The physicians', physiotherapy, and occupational therapy reports do not mention either depression or widespread chronic pain as preventing Ms X from safely climbing stairs. A bungalow is unnecessary for mild TBI. Because she has no objective balance or coordination problems and does not seem to have difficulty recognizing or appropriately responding to emergencies, the proposal is not indicated even if she had a mild–moderate TBI.

   a. It must be noted as well that, according to the occupational therapy records, Ms X was living in a bungalow at the time of the accident, but 2 years later she and her husband purchased and moved into their current 4-story home. She and her husband would have had by that time a clear idea of her situation: well-established and likely permanent impairments and disabilities. There is no history of impulsive behavior. This suggests that a nonmedical rationale may better explain why she purchased and then moved into the current 4-storey home. The proposal is unnecessary.

17. Overall: The plan is seriously flawed, with unjustifiable proposals based on the nature of the original injury and the types of impairments noted in the extant record. Many provisions lack any support from the medical and allied health persons who have assessed or are caring for Ms X. Most other proposals are inapplicable to persons with mild TBI, whereas few would be applicable even if Ms X had indeed had a mild–moderate TBI.

The Person with Amputation and Their Life Care Plan

Robert H. Meier III, MD[a,b,c],*,
Anthony J. Choppa, MEd, CRC, CCM, CDMS[d,e],
Cloie B. Johnson, MEd, ABVE-D, CCM[d,e,f]

KEYWORDS

- Amputation • Life care plan • Prosthetics • Methodology • Standards of practice

KEY POINTS

- The life care planner/case manager relies on the medical community to determine the nature and extent of impairment after a person has had an amputation.
- The life care planner/case manager has specific training in the medical aspects of disability.
- Physical medicine and rehabilitation physicians, also known as physiatrists, provide appropriate medical foundation for recommendations within their scope of practice.
- Prosthetists also may provide medical foundation for recommendations within their scope of practice.
- The life care planner/case managers/physicians focus on the unique rehabilitation needs of the individual patient.

INTRODUCTION

The physiatrist who specializes in rehabilitation of amputees may have experience and expertise to inform the life care planning process.[1] These areas may include the following assessments, therapies, and recommendations:

1. Expectation and changes of function throughout the amputee's life span
2. Potential medical issues that are likely or possibly to be encountered over the lifetime as an amputee

Funding Sources: None to disclose.
Conflict of Interest: None to disclose.
[a] Amputee Services of America, 1601 East 19th Avenue, Suite 3200, Denver, CO 80218, USA; [b] American Academy of Physical Medicine and Rehabilitation, 9700 West Bryn Mawr Avenue, Suite 200, Rosemont, IL 60018-5701, USA; [c] St. Petersburg College, P.O. Box 13489, St. Petersburg, FL 33733-3489, USA; [d] OSC Vocational Systems, Inc, 10132 Northeast 185th Street, Bothell, WA 98011, USA; [e] International Association of Rehabilitation Professionals, 1926 Waukegan Road, Suite 1, Glenview, IL 60025-1770, USA; [f] International Academy of Life Care Planners, 1926 Waukegan Road, Suite 1, Glenview, IL 60025-1770, USA
* Corresponding author.
E-mail address: skipdoc3@gmail.com

Phys Med Rehabil Clin N Am 24 (2013) 467–489
http://dx.doi.org/10.1016/j.pmr.2013.03.004
1047-9651/13/$ – see front matter © 2013 Elsevier Inc. All rights reserved.

3. Most useful prosthetic prescription(s)
4. Frequency of prosthetic replacement (may be in conjunction with the prosthetist)
5. Necessary or useful adaptive equipment
6. Work restrictions given the type(s) of amputation
7. Date most likely that the amputee will achieve maximum medical improvement
8. Types of therapies recommended over the life span, including but not limited to physical therapy, occupational therapy, psychological counseling, vocational rehabilitation, and case management
9. Visits to both the physiatrist and other specialty physicians
10. Life expectancy determination
11. Level of assistance necessary throughout life span
12. Expected emotional adaptation to amputation and the necessity of counseling services with frequency and longevity
13. Pain issues, including potential treatments and prognosis for pain improvement

The life care planner/case manager is part of the multidisciplinary specialty practice of life care planning. The accepted definition of a life care plan and the standards of practice that are published by the International Academy of Life Care Planners (IALCP)[2] are discussed elsewhere in this issue so are not repeated here.

The life care planner/case manager looks to the medical community to define the nature and extent of impairment. The life care planner/case manager does not diagnose or prescribe medical treatment, unless this individual is a physician qualified to do so. The life care planner/case manager has specific training in the medical aspects of disability. The life care planner/case manager has particular expertise in translating the medical implications and prognosis as determined by the physician for a specific patient into recommendations for independent living, employment, and other rehabilitation areas. Specific medical recommendations and many rehabilitation recommendations must come from the medical expert(s), whereas the life care planner/case manager provides recommendations within their specific area of training and knowledge of local resources available and, importantly, the cost of those services and items.

The physiatrist involved in life care plan preparation may also be familiar with local and national trends in prosthetic fitting and the costs of various prostheses. A prosthetist may also be asked to provide a quote for their own prosthetic costs in the life care plan; a physiatrist may be familiar with the costing of prostheses and what costs are locally and nationally.

The life care plan must focus on the needs of the individual patient; the patient and their needs are treated as a unique case study with an n of 1.[3]

Frequently, when a life care plan is coordinated for a patient involved in litigation, courts mandate deadlines and rules of evidence.[4] These deadlines may not be compatible with the patient's having reached maximum medical improvement. In these circumstances, a prognosis from a qualified physician(s) is more critical than ever. However, the standards of practice must be adhered to regardless of any artificially imposed deadline to ensure that proper foundation and methodology are used when preparing the life care plan. The specialized knowledge brought to this collaborative process then ensures a reliable and valid plan, focused on the rehabilitative needs of the individual patient.

The plan resulting from the collaborative process uses both quantitative and qualitative approaches combined with clinical judgment or what is sometimes referred to as experience understood of both the physician and life care planner/case manager.[5] The practitioner's specialized knowledge, grounded in proper methodology within the standards of practice, leads to a realistic and appropriate plan for the patient. The approach is tailored to the needs of the individual and is never akin to a formulaic paint-by-numbers approach. There is no 1 format for the report required. The sample report in this article is for purpose of example only. It is the content, based on sound foundation and accepted methodology, which is important. The life care plan should be supportable, within a degree of reasonable medical probability, regardless whether it is being prepared for the plaintiff or defendant in a litigation case.

The life care plan addresses specific individual needs across several areas. The list shown here is typical, but it is not meant to be exhaustive or all-inclusive.[6]

- Projected evaluations
- Projected treatment needs
- Projected therapeutic modalities
- Medications
- Diagnostics
- Prosthetic needs
- Drug and supply needs
- Orthopedic equipment needs
- Wheelchair and accessories
- Scooter and accessories
- Ergonomic equipment needs
- Aids for independent functioning
- Home modifications
- Home care and residential care
- Leisure, exercise, and recreational equipment
- Future medical and surgical care
- Future medical and surgical risks

Specific treatment needs and prognosis regarding functional outcomes are critical and must be obtained from the physiatrist or other consulting physician specialist(s), as appropriate. Collaboration with the life care planner/case manager regarding realistic and appropriate needs and their coordination is carried out to promote independence in the least restrictive environment with considerations for the patient's safety and dignity.

It is important for the physiatrist involved in life care planning to remember that rehabilitation and function for the person with an amputation are a continuing process. Often, the first prosthesis is not the same prosthesis that will be most appropriate in a year or 2, because the patient's stump likely has changed shaped and lost soft tissue bulk. Also, as the person becomes more adept at prosthetic use, differing components may become more appropriate for subsequent prosthetic restoration. As with stroke or spinal injury patients, what the amputee is able to do 6 months after the amputation is usually less than what the amputee can perform, with subsequent comprehensive rehabilitation, after the amputation. This improvement in function should be anticipated and accounted for in the scope of the life care plan.

Tables 1–19 detail the elements of a hypothetical life care plan that addresses the evaluation, treatment, and rehabilitative needs of an individual who has had a left-knee disarticulation amputation. The tables are provided for purposes of example and to promote education and awareness of the various elements of a life care plan (see **Tables 1–19**).

The IALCP standards of practice[2] require that a proper medical foundation be used when addressing the specific needs of the patient. The standards also require that usual and customary costs be obtained. For patients requiring amputations and

Table 1
Projected evaluations and treatments

Item	Purpose	Provider	Age/Initiated Age/Suspended	Replacement Rate	Base Cost[a]
Amputee clinic (rehabilitation medicine)	Ongoing evaluation, monitoring, and treatment of left-knee disarticulation amputation and sequelae. Address chronic pain issues, surgical recommendations, and future medical and rehabilitation referrals	Local provider	Current age to life expectancy	Average 1–2 visits per year	
Primary care physician evaluation, monitoring, and treatment	Provide preventive care services, screening, health maintenance, and care specifically related to the effects of left-knee disarticulation amputation. Provide treatment recommendations, as needed. Medication management	Local provider	Current age to life expectancy	Average every 6 mo (above and beyond routine needs)	

[a] Base cost should be nondiscounted/market rate prices from verifiable data with referenced sources that are geographically specific when appropriate and available, with more than 1 cost estimate, when appropriate.[7] "Accurate and timely cost information and specificity of service allocations that can be easily used by the client and interested parties" should also be identified.[2]

Table 2
Projected therapeutic modalities

Item	Purpose	Provider	Age/Initiated Age/Suspended	Replacement Rate	Base Cost[a]
Physical therapy evaluation, monitoring, and treatment	Provide therapy with focus on strengthening, stretching, range of motion, and mobility in left lower extremity and knee. Provide gait training as needed, assist with endurance/conditioning with prosthesis related to functional tasks and monitor overuse issues related to hips, knees, and back. Develop individualized structured exercise program	Local provider	Current age to life expectancy	Minimum 1 block of sessions every 5–10 y (10–15 sessions each block)	
Occupational therapy evaluation, monitoring, and treatment	Conduct in-home evaluation to provide equipment/modification recommendations, including bathroom safety as the patient/evaluee ages with disability	Local provider	Current age to life expectancy	2 evaluations total Specific needs pending outcome of each evaluation	
Weight loss program/nutritional counseling	Ongoing evaluation and monitoring of weight in light of left through-the-knee amputation	Local provider	Current age over next 2 y	5 visits	
Individual/family psychological evaluation, monitoring, and treatment	Ongoing evaluation, monitoring, and treatment for emotional adjustment issues related to severe injury and resulting impact on body image, family, familial relationships, and employability	Local provider	Current age to life expectancy	Average weekly sessions for 6–12 mo, then average 1–2 sessions per month for an additional 5 y, then average 12–15 sessions per year for 5 more years. As needed thereafter	

[a] Base cost should be nondiscounted/market rate prices from verifiable data with referenced sources that are geographically specific when appropriate and available, with more than 1 cost estimate, when appropriate.[7] "Accurate and timely cost information and specificity of service allocations that can be easily used by the client and interested parties" should also be identified.[2]

Table 3
Medications

Item (mg)	Purpose	Provider	Age/Initiated Age/Suspended	Replacement Rate	Base Cost[a]
Trazodone[b] (50)	Assist with sleep	Local pharmacy	Current age to life expectancy	Average monthly	
Cymbalta[b] (60)	Management of neuropathic pain	Local pharmacy	Current age to life expectancy	Average monthly	
Deplin[b] (15)	Management of depression	Local pharmacy	Current age to life expectancy	Average monthly	

[a] Base cost should be nondiscounted/market rate prices from verifiable data with referenced sources that are geographically specific when appropriate and available, with more than 1 cost estimate, when appropriate.[7] "Accurate and timely cost information and specificity of service allocations that can be easily used by the client and interested parties" should also be identified.[2]
[b] Reflects current use. Physician may choose to alter dosage or change medication over time.

prostheses, the usual and customary costs are typically the prosthetic laboratory costs listed on an invoice. These costs are not the same as the Medicare allowable reimbursement for the prosthesis or the amount that an insurance company might pay the prosthetic laboratory at a contracted or discounted rate. This situation is in recognition that government or other collateral source funds may change over time because of changes in budgetary policies and may not exist at all in the future. The purpose of the plan is to describe the probable needs and costs of meeting them into the future. The plan must ensure that appropriate funding is available to meet projected needs decades into the future.

Table 4
Diagnostics

Item	Purpose	Provider	Age/Initiated Age/Suspended	Replacement Rate	Base Cost[a]
Radiograph left femur	Monitor amputation site	Local provider	Current age to life expectancy	Average every 5 y	
Radiograph left knee	Monitor amputation site	Local provider	Current age to life expectancy	Average every 5 y	
Radiograph right knee	Monitor right-knee issues related to overuse	Local provider	Current age to life expectancy	Average every 5 y	
Radiograph hips	Evaluate and monitor for arthritis related to injury	Local provider	Current age to life expectancy	Average every 15 y	
Radiograph spine	Evaluate and monitor for spine symptoms related to injury	Local provider	Current age to life expectancy	Average every 15 y	

[a] Base cost should be nondiscounted/market rate prices from verifiable data with referenced sources that are geographically specific when appropriate and available, with more than 1 cost estimate, when appropriate.[7] "Accurate and timely cost information and specificity of service allocations that can be easily used by the client and interested parties" should also be identified.[2]

Table 5
Prosthetic needs: new prostheses

Item	Purpose	Provider	Age/Initiated Age/Suspended	Replacement Rate	Base Cost[a,b]
Knee disarticulation endoskeletal prosthesis base (L5311)	Promote ambulating activities	Local provider	Current age to life expectancy	Average every 4–5 y	$4958.67 each
Above-knee test socket (L5622)	Prosthetic componentry	Local provider	Current age to life expectancy	Average every 4–5 y	$471.69 each
Above-knee acrylic lamination (L5631)	Prosthetic componentry	Local provider	Current age to life expectancy	Average every 4–5 y	$495.39 each
Above-knee total contact (L5650)	Prosthetic componentry	Local provider	Current age to life expectancy	Average every 4–5 y	$647.05 each
Above-knee flexible inner socket/rigid frame (L5651)	Prosthetic componentry	Local provider	Current age to life expectancy	Average every 4–5 y	$1354.01 each
Suction suspension (L5652)	Prosthetic componentry	Local provider	Current age to life expectancy	Average every 4–5 y	$491.56 each
Above-knee alignable system (L5920)	Prosthetic componentry	Local provider	Current age to life expectancy	Average every 4–5 y	$598.22 each
Flex foot system (L5980)	Prosthetic componentry	Local provider	Current age to life expectancy	Average every 4–5 y	$4570.84 each
Ultralight material titanium/carbon (L5950)	Prosthetic componentry	Local provider	Current age to life expectancy	Average every 4–5 y	$1010.71 each
Socks (L8430)	Prosthetic componentry	Local provider	Current age to life expectancy	Average every 2 y	12 at $25.84 each

[a] Base cost should be nondiscounted/market rate prices from verifiable data with referenced sources that are geographically specific when appropriate and available, with more than 1 cost estimate, when appropriate.[7] "Accurate and timely cost information and specificity of service allocations that can be easily used by the client and interested parties" should also be identified.[2]

[b] Costs are noted for educational purposes and reflect 2012 charges for items.

Table 6
C-leg microprocessor knee

Item	Purpose	Provider	Age/Initiated Age/Suspended	Replacement Rate	Base Cost[a]
Single-axis swing and stance knee (L548)	Promote ambulating activities	Local provider	Current age to life expectancy	Average every 4–5 y	$3183.95 each
Stance flexion (L5845)	Prosthetic componentry	Local provider	Current age to life expectancy	Average every 4–5 y	$1983.89 each
Stance extension dampening (L5848)	Prosthetic componentry	Local provider	Current age to life expectancy	Average every 4–5 y	$1190.22 each
Microprocessor control (L5856)	Prosthetic componentry	Local provider	Current age to life expectancy	Average every 4–5 y	$26,570 each
High-activity knee frame (L5930)	Prosthetic componentry	Local provider	Current age to life expectancy	Average every 4–5 y	$3725.57 each
Lithium ion battery (L7368)	Prosthetic componentry	Local provider	Current age to life expectancy	Average every 4–5 y	$558.62 each

[a] Base cost should be nondiscounted/market rate prices from verifiable data with referenced sources that are geographically specific when appropriate and available, with more than 1 cost estimate, when appropriate.[7] "Accurate and timely cost information and specificity of service allocations that can be easily used by the client and interested parties" should also be identified.[2]

Table 7
Socket change

Item	Purpose	Provider	Age/Initiated Age/Suspended	Replacement Rate	Base Cost[a,b]
Replacement socket base (L5701)	Promote ambulating activities	Local provider	Current age to life expectancy	Average every 2–3 y	$5002.90 each
Test socket (L5622)	Prosthetic componentry	Local provider	Current age to life expectancy	Average every 2–3 y	$424.66 each
Acrylic socket (L5631)	Prosthetic componentry	Local provider	Current age to life expectancy	Average every 2–3 y	$495.39 each
Above-knee total contact (L5650)	Prosthetic componentry	Local provider	Current age to life expectancy	Average every 2–3 y	$647.05 each
Above-knee flexible inner socket (L5651)	Prosthetic componentry	Local provider	Current age to life expectancy	Average every 2–3 y	$1354.01 each
Suction suspension (L5652)	Prosthetic componentry	Local provider	Current age to life expectancy	Average every 2–3 y	$491.56 each
Ultralight material titanium/carbon (L5950)	Prosthetic componentry	Local provider	Current age to life expectancy	Average every 2–3 y	$1010.71 each
Socks (L8430)	Prosthetic componentry	Local provider	Current age to life expectancy	Average every 2 y	12 at $25.84 each

[a] Base cost should be nondiscounted/market rate prices from verifiable data with referenced sources that are geographically specific when appropriate and available, with more than 1 cost estimate, when appropriate.[7] "Accurate and timely cost information and specificity of service allocations that can be easily used by the client and interested parties" should also be identified.[2]
[b] Costs are noted for educational purposes and reflect 2012 charges for items.

Table 8
Shower and swimming prosthesis

Item	Purpose	Provider	Age/Initiated Age/Suspended	Replacement Rate	Base Cost[a,b]
Knee disarticulation endoskeletal prosthesis base (L5311)	Shower safety, access to swimming pool, promote overall health, weight management, and maintain and improve strength and agility	Local provider	Current age to life expectancy	Average every 5–10 y	$4958.67 each
Above-knee test socket (L5622)	Prosthetic componentry	Local provider	Current age to life expectancy	Average every 5–10 y	$471.69 each
Above-knee total contact (L5650)	Prosthetic componentry	Local provider	Current age to life expectancy	Average every 5–10 y	$647.05 each
Above-knee alignable system (L5920)	Prosthetic componentry	Local provider	Current age to life expectancy	Average every 5–10 y	$598.22 each
Waterproof single-axis hydraulic knee (L546)	Prosthetic componentry	Local provider	Current age to life expectancy	Average every 5–10 y	$3590.71 each
Manual lock (L5925)	Prosthetic componentry	Local provider	Current age to life expectancy	Average every 5–10 y	$491.72 each
Waterproof foot (L5972)	Prosthetic componentry	Local provider	Current age to life expectancy	Average every 5–10 y	$442 each

[a] Base cost should be nondiscounted/market rate prices from verifiable data with referenced sources that are geographically specific when appropriate and available, with more than 1 cost estimate, when appropriate.[7] "Accurate and timely cost information and specificity of service allocations that can be easily used by the client and interested parties" should also be identified.[2]
[b] Costs are noted for educational purposes and reflect 2012 charges for items.

Table 9
Prosthesis maintenance

Item	Purpose	Provider	Age/Initiated Age/Suspended	Replacement Rate	Base Cost[a]
Gel liners (L5659)	Prosthetic componentry	Local provider	Current age to life expectancy	Average every 9–12 mo	2 at $673.02 each
TES belt (L5695)	Prosthetic componentry	Local provider	Current age to life expectancy	Average annually	$183.87 each
Standard maintenance including foot shell replacement, adjustments, minor repairs	Maintenance to ensure proper operation and fit of prosthetic unit	Local provider	Current age to life expectancy	Average annually	$500 per year
C-leg microprocessor knee	Maintenance to ensure proper operation and fit of prosthetic unit	Local provider	Current age to life expectancy	Average annually	$1000–$1500 per year

[a] Base cost should be nondiscounted/market rate prices from verifiable data with referenced sources that are geographically specific when appropriate and available, with more than 1 cost estimate, when appropriate.[7] "Accurate and timely cost information and specificity of service allocations that can be easily used by the client and interested parties" should also be identified.[2]

Table 10
Drug and supply needs

Item	Purpose	Provider	Age/Initiated Age/Suspended	Replacement Rate	Base Cost[a]
Antifungal cream 12 g (0.42 oz)	Reduce the risk of infection at amputation site	Local provider	Current age to life expectancy	Average every 2–3 mo	
Adaptskin (Adaptlabs, Bainbridge Island, WA, USA)	Maintain skin integrity and minimize hypersensitivity	Local provider	Current age to life expectancy	Average every 6–8 mo	

[a] Base cost should be nondiscounted/market rate prices from verifiable data with referenced sources that are geographically specific when appropriate and available, with more than 1 cost estimate, when appropriate.[7] "Accurate and timely cost information and specificity of service allocations that can be easily used by the client and interested parties" should also be identified.[2]

PATIENT ISSUES
Boney Overgrowth/Heterotopic Ossification

On examination of the residual limb, is there evidence of new bone growth or boney overgrowth? Has this growth been verified by radiograph? Is this bone overgrowth interfering with prosthetic wearing or the comfort of the prosthetic wearing? Is it severe enough that revision surgery should be considered?

Skin Ulcers

Has the amputee experienced skin ulceration in the past or currently? What is the size and severity of these ulcers? Are other skin abnormalities present, such as ingrown hairs?

Pain

Phantom/residual limb/phantom sensation
The presence of pain in the leg or a phantom sensation is not necessarily detrimental or in need of treatment. However, if the phantom pain is frequent or continuous, interferes

Table 11
Orthopedic equipment needs

Item	Purpose	Provider	Age/Initiated Age/Suspended	Replacement Rate	Base Cost[a]
Bilateral crutches (currently using)	Assist in ambulation, particularly when not able to use prosthetic device	Local provider	Current age to life expectancy	Average every 5–7 y	
Front-wheeled walker (currently using)	Assist in ambulation, particularly when not able to use prosthetic device	Local provider	Current age to life expectancy	Average every 5–7 y	

[a] Base cost should be nondiscounted/market rate prices from verifiable data with referenced sources that are geographically specific when appropriate and available, with more than 1 cost estimate, when appropriate.[7] "Accurate and timely cost information and specificity of service allocations that can be easily used by the client and interested parties" should also be identified.[2]

Table 12
Wheelchair and accessories

Item	Purpose	Provider	Age/Initiated Age/Suspended	Replacement Rate	Base Cost[a]
Quickie 2 (SouthwestMedical.com, LLC, Phoenix, AZ, USA) ultralight manual wheelchair[b] with 8-degree back rest bend, adjustable height arms, semipneumatic casters 6 × 1.5, adjustable angle foot plates, rear antitippers, ascent cushion, left amputee support, crutch holder, heavy-duty package	Mobility at home and work when unable to wear prosthesis. Help manage fatigue and fall risks	Local provider	Current age to life expectancy	Average every 5–7 y	
Manual wheelchair maintenance	Maintenance of wheelchair	Local provider	Current age to life expectancy	Average annually	

[a] Base cost should be nondiscounted/market rate prices from verifiable data with referenced sources that are geographically specific when appropriate and available, with more than 1 cost estimate, when appropriate.[7] "Accurate and timely cost information and specificity of service allocations that can be easily used by the client and interested parties" should also be identified.[2]
[b] Reflects current use.

Table 13
Scooter and accessories

Item	Purpose	Provider	Age/Initiated Age/Suspended	Replacement Rate	Base Cost[a]
Power scooter	For long-distance mobility, when unable to wear prosthetic device, fatigued, or when terrain difficulties exist	Local provider	Age 50 y to life expectancy	Average every 8–10 y	
Batteries for power scooter (needs 2)	Power for scooter	Local provider	Age 50 y to life expectancy	Average every 2 y	
Power scooter maintenance	Maintenance of power scooter	Local provider	Age 50 y to life expectancy	Average annually (1–2 h)	
Harmar lift (Harmar, Sarasota, FL, USA) for power scooter	Facilitate transportation of power scooter	Local provider	Age 50 y to life expectancy	Average every 10 y	
Maintenance for lift	Maintain safe operation of equipment	Local provider	Age 50 y to life expectancy	Average annually (1–2 h)	

[a] Base cost should be nondiscounted/market rate prices from verifiable data with referenced sources that are geographically specific when appropriate and available, with more than 1 cost estimate, when appropriate.[7] "Accurate and timely cost information and specificity of service allocations that can be easily used by the client and interested parties" should also be identified.[2]

Table 14
Ergonomic equipment

Item	Purpose	Provider	Age/Initiated Age/Suspended	Replacement Rate	Base Cost[a]
Ergonomic equipment and work station evaluation	Assist with work/educational efforts by assessing for specific equipment needs; specific needs pending outcome of evaluation	Local provider	Current age to life expectancy	Minimum 1 time	
Ergonomic equipment and work station needs	Specific equipment/work station needs pending outcome of evaluation	Local provider	Current age to life expectancy	Pending outcome of evaluation	

[a] Base cost should be nondiscounted/market rate prices from verifiable data with referenced sources that are geographically specific when appropriate and available, with more than 1 cost estimate, when appropriate.[7] "Accurate and timely cost information and specificity of service allocations that can be easily used by the client and interested parties" should also be identified.[2]

Table 15
Aids for independent functioning

Item	Purpose	Provider	Age/Initiated Age/Suspended	Replacement Rate	Base Cost[a]
Bath chair with back (currently using)	Personal hygiene, safety, and self-care in home	Local provider	Current age to life expectancy	Average every 3–5 y	
Hand-held shower (currently using)	Personal hygiene, safety, and self-care in home	Local provider	Current age to life expectancy	Average every 5 y	
Grab bars: 3 (61–91.4 cm) (24–36 inches)	Personal hygiene, safety, and self-care in home	Local provider	Current age to life expectancy	1 time minimum	
Raised toilet seat (currently using the wall and counter for support getting on and off commode)	Personal hygiene, safety, and self-care in home	Local provider	Current age to life expectancy	Average every 5 y	

[a] Base cost should be nondiscounted/market rate prices from verifiable data with referenced sources that are geographically specific when appropriate and available, with more than 1 cost estimate, when appropriate.[7] "Accurate and timely cost information and specificity of service allocations that can be easily used by the client and interested parties" should also be identified.[2]

with prosthetic wearing, limits function, or is poorly tolerated, it should be actively treated. This treatment should be multimodal and not limited to just pain medication.

Treatment
Pain treatment in amputees may best be performed by a physician who understands the cause of pain in amputees. In some geographic locations, this specialty may not

Table 16
Home modifications

Item	Purpose	Provider	Age/Initiated Age/Suspended	Replacement Rate	Base Cost[a]
Barrier-free home	Home modifications for safety and future wheelchair accessibility, including hand rails, ramps, widened doorways, halls, bathroom, kitchen, flooring	Local provider	Current age to life expectancy		

[a] Base cost should be nondiscounted/market rate prices from verifiable data with referenced sources that are geographically specific when appropriate and available, with more than 1 cost estimate, when appropriate.[7] "Accurate and timely cost information and specificity of service allocations that can be easily used by the client and interested parties" should also be identified.[2]

Table 17
Home care and residential care

Item	Purpose	Provider	Age/Initiated Age/Suspended	Replacement Rate	Base Cost[a]
Choreservice worker	Assist with household chores as necessitated by physical condition and physical limitations as a result of knee disarticulation	Local provider	Current age to life expectancy	Number of hours are individualized with consideration for specific limitations and the effects of aging over time	

[a] Base cost should be nondiscounted/market rate prices from verifiable data with referenced sources that are geographically specific when appropriate and available, with more than 1 cost estimate, when appropriate.[7] "Accurate and timely cost information and specificity of service allocations that can be easily used by the client and interested parties" should also be identified.[2]

exist. The pain experienced by amputees is most often related to prosthetic fit issues and may not be amenable to pain medications alone.

The amputation may need to be revised if a magnetic resonance imaging examination reveals a neuroma. Revision may also be necessary if significant skin grafting was performed or if unusual stump contouring has occurred.

Rehabilitation Consideration

Age at onset
It is often suggested that the younger the amputee, the better the function that is attained with rehabilitation. This may be a general myth in rehabilitation. For the older amputee, especially if the amputation resulted from trauma, a return to usual function may occur with a good residual limb, pain control, and integrated rehabilitation services.

Cause: Trauma, Vascular, Burn, Electrical Burn, Oncologic
The cause of the amputation may also affect the functional outcome and quality of life of the patient. If a long period of disability has preceded the amputation, the outcome

Table 18
Leisure, exercise, and recreational equipment

Item	Purpose	Provider	Age/Initiated Age/Suspended	Replacement Rate	Base Cost[a]
Individualized structured exercise program	Promote physical activity, well-being, and weight loss by providing access to exercise equipment in a safe environment. Program developed by physical therapist	Local provider	Current age to life expectancy	Average monthly	

[a] Base cost should be nondiscounted/market rate prices from verifiable data with referenced sources that are geographically specific when appropriate and available, with more than 1 cost estimate, when appropriate.[7] "Accurate and timely cost information and specificity of service allocations that can be easily used by the client and interested parties" should also be identified.[2]

Table 19
Future medical and surgical care

Item	Purpose	Provider	Age/Initiated Age/Suspended	Replacement Rate	Base Cost[a]
Nonsurgical amputation site events	It is probable that the patient/ evaluee will experience skin breakdowns, blisters, and infections that will require emergency room visits, follow-up visits, antibiotic treatment, and a period out of the prosthesis as a result of these probable complications	Local provider	Current age to life expectancy		
Surgical amputation site events	It is probable that the patient/ evaluee will experience a major treatment event requiring hospitalization and surgical intervention, such as amputation site revision, scar revision, debridement, and unresolved infections. Will be out of prosthesis during each event	Local provider	Current age to life expectancy		

[a] Base cost should be nondiscounted/market rate prices from verifiable data with referenced sources that are geographically specific when appropriate and available, with more than 1 cost estimate, when appropriate.[7] "Accurate and timely cost information and specificity of service allocations that can be easily used by the client and interested parties" should also be identified.[2]

may be lessened because of comorbid disease of bones, joints, and muscles in the amputated limb.

Prosthetic Items

Prosthetics/specific components/prices/replacements

Prices for prosthetic devices vary across the United States and Canada. It is essential that the life care plan contain prices that are local and specific to the individual patient.

When considering prosthetic options, it is important to consult with the physiatrist and, when able, the prosthetist regarding specific devices, supplies, backups, and other items. The life care plan included in this article exemplifies the various components that may be considered.

Durable Medical Equipment

Gait aids

Items such as canes, crutches, and walkers may be appropriate inclusions in this category.

Again, the specific needs of the patient must be considered.

Wheelchair: manual/powered/scooter

The need for a wheelchair in patients with lower extremity amputation can be a source of misunderstanding. Accordingly, wheelchair use must be considered within the specific situation of an individual and their life. It may be that an individual is expected to be functional at work or in other life roles, such as parent, on days when they cannot wear their prosthetic device because of broken components or a problem anatomically. Regardless, they may be required to fulfill their obligations as a worker, spouse, parent, and so forth. The individual must carry on with life. Therefore, a wheelchair may be required when a person is unable to wear a prosthetic device because of such complications as skin irritations, ulcers, ingrown hairs, or abrasions on the amputation site. Further, it is not uncommon that a person experiencing amputation chooses to use a wheelchair in the home for a reprieve from walking or in using the prosthesis or other gait aides. Longer-distance ambulation and ease in getting to or from the bathroom at night are other functions for which a wheelchair can provide appropriate assistance. The life care planner must consider the big picture of the patient's life now and into the future.

Recommendation for a power wheelchair or scooter carries some additional costs for the transportation of the device. Powered wheelchairs typically require a fully modified van with a lift because of the equipment's weight. However, when use of a scooter is appropriate, it can be transported with a simpler adaptive aide attached to most vehicle makes and models. A sample of a device for transporting a scooter, (a Harmar lift) is included in **Table 13**.

FUTURE MEDICAL NEEDS
Low Back Pain

Findings in the literature support an onset of biomechanical low back pain in many patients who have had lower extremity amputation and who have used their prosthetic devices over time. It is appropriate for the life care plan to identify future needs in this regard to provide for appropriate assessment and treatment.

When preparing the life care plan, the following medical assessment form may be used (**Box 1**).

Box 2 lists expected functional outcomes for most amputees with a particular common level of amputation. This checklist is most useful by indicating "Yes" or "No" before each listed item of function. If the amputee is not capable of performing a given function, the reason for not being able to do so should be stated.

Specific functional outcomes are unique to the individual patient. The functions outlined in **Box 2** reflect general guidelines and indicators only.

Vocational Considerations

The individuality of each patient must be taken into account, considering their age, education, work history, transferable skills, interests, achievement and aptitude test results, and other life roles when addressing work. A qualified rehabilitation counselor can perform a vocational assessment with recommendations from the physician regarding physical capabilities. A specific and tailored vocational rehabilitation plan may be necessary if the individual cannot return to their usual and customary

Box 1
Initial rehabilitation medicine evaluation
Date
Name
Date of birth
Date of onset
Referral source
History of present problem
Handedness
Prosthetist
Current prosthesis and its use
Prior prosthetics
Prosthetic training and therapies in the past
Rehabilitation history
Inpatient
Outpatient
Team members
Review of symptoms
Pain
Other systems affected from illness or injury
Past medical history
Smoking
Alcohol
Weight
Medications
Allergies
Vocation
Avocation
Education (school)
Family history
Psychosocial history
Sexual function
Appetite
Sleep
Physical examination
Ambulation history
Medical record review
Level of function and 24-hour typical day
Wheelchair
Gait aids

Driving

Adaptive equipment

Living environment

Impression (diagnoses)

Clinical comments

Recommendations

Photographs and date taken

Location where photographs were taken

---

occupation, or if the individual has had an amputation at a young age before completing school and entering the workforce.

Personal Assistance

It is likely that providing some personal assistance to an amputee decreases the burden placed on the individual's remaining extremities and may prevent overuse problems in the future. Recommendations from the physician regarding physical capabilities and overuse issues are critical in assessing this need. When necessary, the life care planner/case manager can perform specific assessments in the individual's home considering current or future life roles and demands. For example, is the individual a young mother with an infant? Is the individual a middle-aged man working in a heavy industrial trade? These types of considerations have an impact on the need for and amount of assistance that is appropriate to maintain balance between the patient's life roles. We all wear many hats in our lives. We may be workers, students, parents, sons, daughters, men, women, home owners, sports coaches, church members, and so forth. Balance between all life roles is critical, and 1 of the goals of the life care plan is to achieve such balance.

Transportation

It is probable that an individual with an amputation will be able to drive after proper assessment for vehicle modifications and safety response time. The modifications may be simple, such as a steering wheel knob, or may be more complex, such as total hand controls. Other comorbidities affecting function may affect driving after amputation. Recommendation for a driving evaluation by a qualified occupational therapist should be considered when appropriate to ensure the safety of both the driver and the general public.

Longevity

Some findings in the literature suggest that the life span of an amputee may be shorter than that of a nonamputee. However, the studies in question that make this suggestion were performed on an amputee population of older, dysvascular persons in the Veterans Administration system. If the person for whom the life care plan is being prepared is a younger person who was previously healthy and has no significant comorbidities, it is likely the individual will have a normal life span.

Changes Over the Life Span

Changes that occur with aging affect everyone; however, aging with an amputation may contribute to the early onset of decreased abilities. Aging with disability within

Box 2
Expected functional outcomes

Transtibial Level
Increased energy expenditure of 25%–45% more than normal

Yes   No

1. Ambulation with prosthesis on all surfaces
2. No gait aids
3. Independent in donning and doffing prosthesis
4. Standing, up to 2 continuous hours
5. Walking, up to 2 continuous hours
6. Gets up from kneeling
7. Return to recreational activities (eg, hunting, fishing, golfing, jogging, skiing), if performed before amputation
8. Return to previous work
9. Comfortable with falling techniques
10. Performs cardiovascular conditioning program safely
11. Drives
12. Shops
13. Performs housework, gardening, home maintenance
14. Independent in activities of daily living
15. Knows how to purchase correct footwear
16. Can inspect skin and nails for remaining foot
17. Ascends and descends stairs step over step
18. Can run (if patient desires and has adequate cardiopulmonary reserve)

Transfemoral
Increased energy expenditure of 65%–100% more than normal

Yes   No

1. Ambulation with prosthesis on all surfaces
2. No gait aids
3. Independent in donning and doffing prosthesis
4. Standing, up to 2 continuous hours
5. Walking, up to 2 continuous hours
6. Gets up from kneeling
7. Return to recreational activities (eg, hunting, fishing, golfing, jogging, skiing), if performed before amputation
8. Return to previous work
9. Comfortable with falling techniques
10. Performs cardiovascular conditioning program safely
11. Drives
12. Shops
13. Performs housework, gardening, home maintenance
14. Independent in activities of daily living

15. Knows how to purchase correct footwear

16. Can inspect skin and nails on remaining foot

17. Ascends and descends stairs 1 step at a time usually

18. Can run (if patient desires and has adequate cardiopulmonary reserve)

Transradial

Yes   No

1. Independent in donning and doffing prosthesis

2. Independent in activities of daily living

3. Writes legibly with remaining hand

4. Has switched hand dominance, if necessary

5. Drives

6. Can tie laces with 1 hand

7. Uses a button hook easily

8. Has prepared a meal

9. Has been evaluated for adaptive equipment for kitchen and activities of daily living

10. Has performed home and auto maintenance, if appropriate

11. Wears prosthesis during all waking hours

12. Uses prosthesis for most bimanual activities

13. Has returned to same or modified work

Transhumeral

Yes   No

1. Independent in donning and doffing prosthesis

2. Independent in activities of daily living

3. Writes legibly with remaining hand

4. Has switched hand dominance, if necessary

5. Drives

6. Can tie laces with 1 hand

7. Uses a button hook easily

8. Has prepared a meal

9. Has been evaluated for adaptive equipment for kitchen and activities of daily living

10. Has performed home and auto maintenance, if appropriate

11. Wears prosthesis during all waking hours

12. Uses prosthesis for most bimanual activities

13. Has returned to same or modified work

the population with spinal cord injury is a topic of research and publication. It has been suggested that 20 to 30 years after the onset of the disability, premature aging or degeneration occurs. For a person with lower extremity amputation, for example, the life care planner may need to address the onset of low back pain or early onset of degenerative joint disease. Upper extremity amputation may involve overuse of the nonaffected extremity or joints above the level of amputation.

SUMMARY

When coordinating a life care plan, it is critical that proper medical foundation be established. Further, the goal of the life care plan is to promote independence with considerations for safety and human dignity. An individual who has sustained amputation is challenged in these areas. To accomplish this goal, the life care plan must focus on the individual and their unique current and future life circumstances.

REFERENCES

1. Weed R, Sluis A. Life care plans for the amputee: a step by step guide. Boca Raton (FL): CRC Press; 1990.
2. International Academy of Life Care Planners. Standards of practice for life care planners. J Life Care Plan 2006;5(3):75–81.
3. Choppa A, Johnson C. Response to estimating earning capacity: venues, factors and methods. Estimating Earning Capacity: A Journal of Debate and Discussion 2008;1(1):41–2.
4. Weed R, Johnson C. Life care planning in light of Daubert and Kumho. Athens (GA): Elliott & Fitzpatrick; 2006.
5. Choppa A, Johnson C, Shafer LK, et al. The efficacy of professional clinical judgment: developing expert testimony in cases involving vocational rehabilitation and care planning issues. J Life Care Plan 2004;3(3):131–50.
6. Weed R, Berens D, editors. Life care planning and case management handbook. 3rd edition. Boca Raton (FL): St Lucie/CRC Press; 2010.
7. Preston K, Johnson C. Consensus and majority statements derived from life care planning summits held in 2000, 2002, 2004, 2006, 2008, 2010 and 2012. J Life Care Plan 2012;11(2):9–14.

Life Care Planning for the Child with Cerebral Palsy

Richard T. Katz, MD[a],*, Cloie B. Johnson, MEd, ABVE-D, CCM[b,c]

KEYWORDS

- Life expectancy • Cerebral palsy • Life care planning

KEY POINTS

- Life expectancy is reduced in individuals with all but the mildest forms of cerebral palsy.
- Life care plans need to consider what services are reasonably available now and in the future.
- Life care planners need to have experience in treating patients with cerebral palsy, and in evaluating what therapeutic treatments, drugs, procedures, and exposures have proven value.
- Ongoing assistive/nursing care is the most costly item in the life care plan, and numerous factors influence decisions about future caregiving.

INTRODUCTION

Physicians may be asked to help plan for the long-term needs of children with cerebral palsy. Their role may be as a life care planner or in collaboration with a life care planner as described in the article by Johnson and Weed elsewhere in this issue. One of the keys to constructing successful life care plans is to be intimately familiar with the needs of the child with cerebral palsy. It requires extensive experience and training to plan accurately for the needs of an impaired child.

Children with cerebral palsy are often grouped into 4 categories: spastic (approximately 70%), athetoid (approximately 20%), ataxic (approximately 10%), and mixed. Spastic syndromes are most common and are characterized by muscular hypertonicity and loss of motor control. Spastic syndromes may affect predominantly 1 side (hemiplegia), both legs (paraplegia), legs greater than arms (diplegia), or all 4 limbs (quadriplegia or tetraplegia). Athetoid or dyskinetic syndromes are characterized by

Funding Sources: None to disclose.
Conflict of Interest: None to disclose.
[a] Washington University School of Medicine, 4660 Maryland Avenue, Suite 250, St Louis, MO 63108, USA; [b] OSC Vocational Systems, Inc, 10132 Northeast 185th Street, Bothell, WA 98011, USA; [c] International Academy of Life Care Planners/International Association of Rehabilitation Professionals, 1926 Waukegan Road, Suite 1, Glenview, IL 60025-1770, USA
* Corresponding author.
E-mail address: pianodoctor@pol.net

slow writhing, involuntary movements, and sometimes abrupt, distal, jerky movements. Ataxic syndromes are uncommon ($\sim 10\%$) and may be marked by weakness, incoordination, wide-based gait, and tremor. Many patients have mixed features.

A recent consensus group[1] defined cerebral palsy as an "umbrella term covering a group of non-progressive, but often changing, motor impairment syndromes secondary to lesions or anomalies of the brain arising in the early stages of its development." Recent studies suggest that cerebral palsy is a common cause of childhood disability, with significant associated disability. More than 100,000 Americans younger than 18 years are believed to have some neurologic disability attributed to cerebral palsy.[2] Approximately 25% of children with cerebral palsy in France and England cannot walk, and 30% are classified as mentally retarded.[3,4] A simple examination of these statistics suggests that health care practitioners and the social community need to plan for the survival and care for those within this population.

Life Care Planning

When planning the lifelong needs for a child, a life care plan may be constructed. A life care plan estimates what services are necessary and appropriate to meet the coordination of future medical and rehabilitation services and the costs associated to promote quality of life in the least restrictive environment with respect for independence and human dignity. When constructing a life care plan, it first must be determined what is the nature and extent of any impairment, including the physical, emotional, or cognitive impairments noted during the course of evaluation and the expected outcome over time. Although the entire process of life care planning is articulated in greater length elsewhere in this issue, **Box 1** summarizes its steps.

A physician with experience assessing and treating children with cerebral palsy can give increasingly accurate estimates of a child's prognosis for improvement during serial observations of the child's developmental areas: gross motor skills, fine motor and adaptive skills, personal and social skills, speech and language skills, and cognitive and emotional development. With this knowledge, a life care plan can be developed to assess the needs and benefits of future medical treatments and rehabilitation interventions (eg, physical therapy, occupational therapy, and speech therapy).

To formulate the lifetime costs, it is necessary to estimate the life expectancy of the child, which has been a source of considerable debate. This topic is reviewed in some depth later. The physician and life care planner with proper foundation must estimate the need, duration of need, and costs for a wide variety of hardware items and services. Examples of such devices include wheelchairs, seating systems, orthopedic aids, orthotics, home furnishings, architectural modifications and aids for independent function, drugs, supplies, and leisure-time equipment. The child's future home or facility care costs can similarly be approximated by planning for the appropriate level of daily care (eg, home aid, skilled care within the home, or care provided by a children's home occupant). The life care costs must include services rendered by physical, occupational, and speech therapists, and other educational and psychological services. Costs for future medical and surgical care, and the costs of potential future medical complications and procedures, must be appraised.

Services Reasonably Available Now and in the Future

Life care planning standards of practice articulate the need for using reasonably available resources. It is important to understand the limitations on any resources and their expected availability into the future. Planning for children with cerebral palsy often involves a variety of sources, including social services, because children

Box 1
Steps in the formation of a life care plan

1. Determine extent and sequelae of the child's physical, emotional, or cognitive impairments
2. Estimate prognosis
3. Estimate the need for and benefit of further medical and rehabilitative interventions
4. Determine the additional items required for long-term care. Categories to be considered within a life care plan include the following:

    a. Projected evaluations

    b. Projected therapeutic modalities

    c. Diagnostic testing/educational assessment

    d. Wheelchair needs

    e. Wheelchair accessories and maintenance

    f. Aids for independent functioning

    g. Orthotics/prosthetics

    h. Home furnishings and accessories

    i. Drug/supply needs

    j. Home care/facility care

    k. Future medical care (routine)

    l. Transportation

    m. Health and strength maintenance

    n. Architectural renovations

    o. Potential complications

    p. Future medical care/surgical intervention or aggressive treatment

    q. Orthopedic equipment needs

    r. Vocational/educational plan

5. The final step is to identify the costs for the medical and rehabilitative services, equipment, supplies, and services

with physical and mental handicaps have a variety of psychosocial challenges related to their impairments. A discussion of these challenges is beyond the scope of this article, but interested readers are referred to other sources for further inquiry.[5] However, it is useful to be aware of what types of social support services are available within the locality of the disabled child and any limitations or guarantees they may hold.

Estimating Life Expectancy

As discussed earlier, one of the key issues in creating a robust life care plan is to provide an estimate of life expectancy. A considerable amount of epidemiologic literature has provided guidance in this regard. However, such literature is often left unexamined by parties when determining or negotiating future costs. This literature is reviewed as it applies to children with cerebral palsy and mental retardation. As a preface to this analysis, the interface between scientific and legal thought is addressed. One of the important issues in bridging the gap between physicians and attorneys in this regard relates to the issue of what constitutes a fact. As described by Taylor[6]:

> Health care providers tend to view facts as being those observations which are based upon empirical evaluation. For a fact to be accepted as true it usually must be confirmed with certainty. On the other hand, for lawyers involved in civil litigation, facts are established by the legal construct of probability. Thus, even in the absence of complete scientific certainty, a legal fact is deemed to be true, if the observation is more likely than not found to be correct.

This discrepancy in what constitutes a fact is a key source of miscommunication between lawyer and physician.[7] The physician needs to understand that litigation holds to a standard of "more likely than not" or "less likely than not." Another often-used phrase is "within the realm of medical certainty." In the legal sense, this phrase simply means that the probability that a fact is true is greater than 50%. With this construct in mind, the following epidemiologic studies have been summarized (when possible) to address the following important question: "When is it more likely than not that a child with cerebral palsy or mental retardation will no longer be alive?"

Life expectancy of those with cerebral palsy has been well studied, and yet this literature has been at times distorted and manipulated when presented in scientific testimony. This literature has been extensively reviewed, and readers are referred to these articles for more exhaustive review.[8,9] Presented in the following sections is a summary of some of the key points.

Some life care planners use a normal life expectancy for children with cerebral palsy. Is that appropriate?

Except for children with the mildest cerebral palsy, it is clearly erroneous to state that life expectancy is normal. In an article published in the New England Journal of Medicine in 1990,[9] Eyman and colleagues reported on 99,543 persons with developmental disability from the California Department of Developmental Services. The best predictors of mortality were (1) deficits in cognitive function, (2) limitations on mobility, (3) incontinence, and (4) inability to eat without assistance. These investigators provided a life table analysis of survival, based on defining 3 subgroups of children:

Subgroup 1: immobile, not toilet trained, required tube feeding
Subgroup 2: immobile, not toilet trained, but could eat with assistance
Subgroup 3: mobile but not ambulatory and could eat with assistance

Subsequently, a significant error in data manipulation in Eyman and colleagues'[10] study was pointed out, resulting in life expectancies that were too low. The corrected life table for subgroups 1, 2, and 3 is shown in **Table 1**.

This was the first of many articles in the medical literature that reported a reduction in life expectancy for most persons with cerebral palsy.

What factors are important in predicting cerebral palsy?

The life span of the child with cerebral palsy is curtailed by the presence of certain key disabilities, summarized in **Box 2**. Decreased cognitive abilities are associated with diminished life span, even in the absence of physical impairment. Generally, life expectancy for physically and mentally disabled persons has increased compared with life expectancies from many decades ago, but generally not in the past 10 to 20 years.

The findings in the medical literature with respect to life expectancy and cerebral palsy are consistent. One of the key problems in comparing survival in different population groups of children with cerebral palsy is comparing prognosis in children with

Table 1
Survival in 3 groups of developmentally disabled children (corrected data)

Age	Subgroup 1: % Surviving to Age Interval	Subgroup 1: Life Expectancy (y)	Subgroup 2: % Surviving to Age Interval	Subgroup 2: Life Expectancy (y)	Subgroup 3: % Surviving to Age Interval	Subgroup 3: Life Expectancy (y)
1	100	11.2	100	25.0	100	42.7
5	66	12.2	85	25.2	95	40.9
10	41	13.1	67	26.2	89	38.5
15	27	13.7	54	26.9	82	36.4
20	18	14.6	45	26.7	77	33.8
25	13	14.8	39	25.7	71	31.6
30	9	14.6	34	23.9	66	28.6
35	6	14.6	30	21.6	62	25.4
40	5	13.3	27	19.1	58	22.1
45	4	12.1	24	16.2	53	18.9
50	3	9.4	21	13.1	46	16.1
55	2	7.5	16	11.5	38	14.2
60	1	6.3	11	10.2	31	11.6
65	<1	4.7	7	9.1	25	9.1
70	<1	3.6	5	7.8	15	8.3
75	<1	4.0	3	6.3	10	6.0
80	<1	2.5	1	6.6	4	7.1
85	<1	2.5	<1	4.0	3	3.3

Data from Life Expectancy for CP, VS, TBI and SCI. Correction of Eyman et al. (1990) life expectancies. Available at: http://www.lifeexpectancy.com/eyman.shtml. Accessed August 19, 2012.

similar severity of disability. Some investigators chose more broad categories of disability and others more narrow ones, complicating the analysis. However, subsequent reanalysis of data using similar categories of disability show marked homogeneity in outcomes.[8,11]

Are there opinions contrary to the mainstream in the cerebral palsy survival literature?
The cerebral palsy survival literature contains some data that vary markedly from the balance of the literature. In 1998, a study was published of 371 children with cerebral palsy in 3 registered nurse (RN)-staffed nursing facilities in the Chicago area.[12] This study divided its study population into groups based on functional abilities in the manner of Eyman[9] to compare statistical results. Survival rates for groups 1 to 4 were notably longer, reaching both statistical as well as clinical significance. The study population was small; only 251 children had significant mental impairment and cerebral palsy. The number of children in groups 4, 5, and 6 were only 11, 9, and 2, respectively. The study population was all inpatient, a notable distinction to the thousands of patients in the California cohort. Details of the data analysis were not provided, leaving the reader uninformed as to the statistical methods used.

Subsequently, it was shown that a X^2 method was used to analyze the data, a type of statistical test that is not appropriate for a survival analysis. The article was rejected by the *American Journal of Children* because of statistical problems.[13] Furthermore, the subject count seems confusing: at 1 point, 371 children are reported to have

---

Box 2
Key disabilities diminishing life expectancy in children with cerebral palsy

- Presence and severity of mental retardation
- Inability to speak intelligible words
- Inability to recognize voices
- Inability to interact with peers
- Physical disability
- Limitations on mobility
- Inability to propel wheelchair
- Inability to roll over
- Inability to creep/crawl/scoot
- Lack of upper extremity function
- Inability to eat without assistance
- Tube feeding
- Incontinence
- Cortical blindness
- Presence and severity of seizures
  - Is the medical literature consistent in its findings?

---

cerebral palsy, yet later in the paper only 367 had. In deposition testimony, the principal author mentioned that patients with developmental disability comprised 31 of the patients, and none had cerebral palsy. The article did not consider the many studies included in topical reviews,[8] instead concentrating only on Eyman's studies. The study did not note any difference in outcome of children with tracheostomy, in contrast with other studies in the literature.[14] Despite its flaws, the article supports the role of severity of mental retardation, presence and severity of epilepsy, and the importance of arm movement/mobility/rolling as important factors in predicting survival. The choice of journal for publication is questionable, because the publication is outside the literature arena of most people interested in this topic.

The same author[15] published a follow-up study that extended observations to 447 children. Both articles suffer from statistical flaws that ensure that the survival probabilities were too high.[10,16,17] The errors are 2-fold: (1) the author did not use a standard survival analysis and instead relied on an incorrect method of his own; and (2) in comparing his own work with Eyman's, the author used the erroneous data published in Eyman's original *New England Journal of Medicine* article,[9] which provided overly pessimistic longevity figures because of a mathematical error, instead of the corrected data (see **Table 1**).[10]

Has there been any improvement in life expectancy in children with cerebral palsy over the last 30 years?

Some data show that children in some subgroups of cerebral palsy are living longer. Investigators following a longitudinal cohort of children with cerebral palsy sought to determine whether there were changes in survival within their population (47,259 persons with cerebral palsy receiving services from the State of California) between 1983 and 2002.[17] In children with cerebral palsy who had severe disabilities, and in adults who required gastrostomy feeding, the investigators found an improvement in life expectancy. Life expectancies reported in earlier studies should be increased by approximately 5 years based on the most recent mortality data. Although survival of these most fragile children improved, no significant increase in life expectancy was seen in other subgroups.

This finding corresponds closely with findings from a group of investigators from Israel who sought to identify risk factors for early childhood mortality with cerebral palsy.[18] One thousand children sequentially referred to 1 development center were followed for more than 20 years. Eighty-one children died, and they were compared with 81 age-matched controls, and 81 developmentally disabled children without neurologic deficits. The principal findings were that (1) children with a lack of mobility or nonindependent feeding had a life expectancy into their mid-teens, and (2) socioeconomic variables were not associated with life expectancy.

Investigators from Sweden studied survival in children with cerebral palsy followed over 15 years.[19] Survival status was known for 99.3% of the whole study population with cerebral palsy, a study strength. The estimated survival was 60% at age 19 years in children with the most severe gross motor limitations, as assessed by the Gross Motor Functional Classification System V (GMFCSV) and who required a percutaneous endoscopic gastrostomy (PEG) tube. GMFCSV indicates children who have the most severe motor deficit. Children with milder forms of cerebral palsy had considerably greater longevity. Gastrostomy tube feeding was associated with a 9-fold increased risk of dying, regardless of GMFCSV level. No difference in mortality was seen between boys and girls.

Australian investigators reported on the survival of individuals with cerebral palsy between 1970 and 2004.[20] Individuals with cerebral palsy had an 80% survival rate to the age of 40 years. The inability to ambulate independently was the strongest predictor of mortality. Compared with those with mild motor impairment, the mortality risk of those with severe motor impairment was 30 times higher. In those with severe motor impairment, survival was determined by the number of additional impairments, including epilepsy, severe/profound intellectual impairment, blindness, deafness, and lack of speech. Consistent with previous findings in the literature, the most severely impaired children had life expectancies of 21 years. Thirty-five percent survived 30 years. Gastrostomy tube use was not presented. Confirming work of others,[17] no improvement in survival was seen in the 30 years between the 1970s and 2000s.

Data from children with cerebral palsy in California and Sweden have been compared[21] and provide additional evidence that survival probabilities are remarkably similar for severely disabled children in developed countries. As reported by the study investigators, "this may suggest that there are not major differences in the type and quality of care delivered in these countries."

Is cognitive impairment without physical impairment associated with shorter life expectancy?

Life expectancy in children with developmental disability, but with normal physical function, has been well studied over the last 50 years. Diminution of life expectancy is strongly related to the severity of developmental disability. Recent studies continue to show this relationship. Two thousand three hundred and sixty-six persons from the Finnish Population Register Center were followed since 1962, with a mean follow-up of 26.9 years.[22] For persons with mild developmental disability, life expectancy did not differ from the general population. In the group with moderate developmental disability, the decrement was slight, but in the severe and profoundly disabled groups, a 19% to 35% diminishment in life expectancy was observed.

Other researchers[23] have found median life expectancies of 74.0, 67.6, and 58.6 years, respectively, for people with mild, moderate, and severe levels of handicap. Another group[24] assessed excess mortality in persons with intellectual disability (non-Down and Down syndrome) compared with the general population. All-cause and disease-specific mortality were approximately 3 times higher in these groups than in the general population. The most profound differences were noted in persons in their third decade: all-cause mortality was about 9 times higher in men and about 17 times higher in women. In the group excluding those with Down syndrome, both males and females had a standardized mortality ratio of almost 3.0.

What is the life expectancy for children with cerebral palsy?

The life expectancy literature for children with cerebral palsy shows that children with mild cerebral palsy have a normal or near-normal life expectancy. Children with the most profound cerebral palsy have a life expectancy of 19 to 21 years. Intermediate degrees of severity of neurologic deficit are associated with intermediate life expectancy.

Life Care Planning Issues

The following discussion covers topics related to key ethical and decision-making processes in the life care plan for the child with cerebral palsy. Routine items such as the cost of a wheelchair and how it can be amortized over 3 to 5 years require no special discussion in this article. A hypothetical case is used as an example.

RBK is a 5-year-old boy with severe developmental delay after an anoxic/hypoxic encephalopathy that occurred after cardiopulmonary arrest on October 3, 2008, when he was approximately 6 months of age. His deficits include a severe uncontrolled seizure disorder, severe mental retardation and global developmental delays, oculomotor dysfunction resulting in bilateral medial rectus recessions, and spastic tetraparesis (worse on the left). He has no functional grasp, rolling, crawling, sitting, or head control. He speaks no words. It is not clear that he recognizes voices or faces. He requires a gastronomy tube for all nutrition and medication administration.

What are the initial factors for consideration?

After evaluating the nature and extent of the impairment, the life care plan was opined to be based on a life expectancy to 19 to 21 years, in accordance with findings in the literature presented earlier. In the process of litigation, the expert witness was asked to make a best estimate of future life expectancy. Because there is no crystal ball, the best estimate can be made by systematically reviewing the literature discussed earlier applied to the individual patient.

In terms of expenses, the 3 most important factors for any life care plan are (1) the amount of years surviving; (2) the amount, duration, and intensity of long-term care (ie, nursing services); and (3) the amount, frequency, and duration of therapy services. Thus, each of these factors should have an extensive justification.

What factors play in the estimation of future costs?

The International Academy of Life Care Planners standards of practice specifically outline the basic components and process for life care planning. The methodology remains consistent, although individual differences may present themselves. Within certain diagnoses, as described earlier, there are also consistent areas of impairment. Factors that may remain variable include analysis of the individual patient. Although the life care planning process should be objective and attend to the needs of the child, in litigation there may be opposite views or at least diverse plaintiff and defense views. Although it may be difficult for the novice to envision an appropriate life care plan for the child's lifetime, it should be pointed out that the life care planner generally has but 1 opportunity to develop a plan (ie, if provisions are not included in the original life care plan, they likely will never be addressed again). What level of care should the life care planner provide for? The short answer is the level of care that is necessary and appropriate to meet the coordination of future medical and rehabilitation services to promote quality of life in the least restrictive environment with respect for independence and human dignity. It may be found in the litigation process that advocacy of the plaintiff and defendant may create a faux friction point regarding this issue. The standards of practice must be used as written, as published in peer-reviewed journals, and generally accepted within the international community of life care planners. The following comments are addressed by common categories within the life care plan.

Projected evaluations Routine physical therapy, occupational therapy, speech, and other evaluations are typical in the life care plan of any person with substantial disability. Typically, children receive a yearly evaluation as part of their individualized educational plan within the school system; however, this is limited in scope to what is educationally appropriate. The life care planner may ask whether a child's school has a reasonable program for children with developmental disability. Are adjuvant physical, occupational, and speech therapy evaluations necessary in addition to what is offered within the school system? Is a vocational evaluation necessary if a child could never be competitively employed? How long does the school system provide rehabilitation services – until 21 years (most states) or later (Michigan)? This situation may require evaluation beyond any school's review to ensure that all areas of life are addressed.

Projected therapeutic modalities
In life care plans for children with cerebral palsy, the plan is often front-loaded with physical, occupational, and speech therapy. The life care planner should ensure that the plan is realistic in the implementations. If physical therapy, occupational therapy, speech-language pathology, and other therapies are recommended twice per week beyond school needs, little time may be available to successfully implement these therapies within the course of a day. At times, these additional therapies may substitute for the academic curriculum. The life care plan also requires appropriate foundation. Studies in adults with brain injury suggest that persons with moderate neurologic deficit benefit the most, whereas those with profound or minimal deficits less so.[25] The life care planner should consider several issues: what is the evidence that therapies benefit children with cerebral palsy? Are therapy visits needed to supplement what is already provided within the school system? How many visits are needed? Do children with different severities of cerebral palsy have benefit, whereas others little to none? Are therapies necessary to maintain function so that it does not decline?

Physical therapy is typically started early in life in children with cerebral palsy and then continued by parents within the home.[26] The parent's ability to provide therapy in the home can be affected by several factors. Such factors require analysis, including the health of the parents, the number of siblings the child with cerebral palsy has, and the parent's employment status. Investigators have suggested that therapy continue to age 12 or 14 years, after which the child plateaus and therapeutic goals are integrated into daily activities. In 1 study the investigators compared 48 infants 12 to 19 months in age who were randomly assigned to either 12 months of physical therapy or 6 months of infant stimulation followed by 6 months of physical therapy. The purely physical therapy group fared more poorly, and significant differences between groups persisted after 12 months. No significant difference was seen in the need for bracing or orthopedic surgery.[27]

Family and individual counseling is another area of consideration. Life care planners may include extensive funds for counseling within the life care plan without due thought or consideration. Investigators[28] have studied patterns in psychotherapy and noted that the average number of sessions is 8. The average number of sessions required to see improvement in about half of patients with depression/anxiety is 13 to 18, and the most dramatic improvement is seen between sessions 7 and 10. Again, individual assessment with appropriate foundation is required. The life care plan is not a theoretic construct.

Diagnostic testing and schooling

The life care planner needs to determine if a reasonable school experience is available within the child's district, or if another educational/care experience needs to be considered. The adequacy of school systems to meet the needs of the disabled child is the subject of considerable controversy and litigation, which are outside the scope of this article.

The need for ongoing neuropsychological assessment of the child with cerebral palsy may be a routine part of the individualized educational plan, or it may not be performed routinely and needs to be assessed separately. However, although neuropsychological testing is undoubtedly useful, it can be overused and its applicability in real-world settings may be questioned.[29] Consideration of the reasonableness and purpose of routine testing is needed. Is routine testing being completed to assess progress? Is it to aid in developing compensatory strategies?

Wheelchairs, facilitative devices, orthopedic equipment

Costs of durable medical goods are rarely the subject of significant debate. The need for an electric wheelchair is generally based on the child's physical ability to operate a joystick or similar mechanical interface, and requires the cognitive ability to navigate the chair within their environment. Replacement schedules and amortization of such devices are covered elsewhere in this issue. Many experienced rehabilitation professionals have ongoing records from their clinical practice for appropriate contacts for goods and services for persons with disability, assembled after many years of research. Although the Internet provides ready access to goods, services, and costs, case managers and life care planners are the professionals who work directly with medical and rehabilitation cost identification. They are continuously researching the costs for current and future medical and rehabilitation treatment and services, equipment and other needs. These professionals understand the intricacies of medical billing practices. Although physicians have understanding within their practice, they may, if completing a life care plan themselves, request the services of an individual with this particular expertise.

Drugs and supply needs

Similarly, the costs of medications and disposable medicals should be identified primarily by the current provider of these drugs and supplies. The Life Care Planning Summit of 2012 held in Dallas, Texas resulted in the following consensus statement with respect to drug and supply costs:

- Verifiable data from appropriately referenced sources
- Costs identified are geographically specific when appropriate and available
- Nondiscounted/market rate prices
- More than 1 cost estimate, when appropriate

Life care planners should use generic medication costs when available. Although the price of a particular drug may be reduced substantially when the drug loses proprietary status and becomes generic, this may not provide a good estimate of future drug costs, because new proprietary drugs may be introduced at higher prices.

Home and facility care

The costs of home and facility care are the largest budget item in a life care plan and may not be fully discussed and justified. The Life Care Planning Summit of 2010, held in Atlanta, Georgia resulted in the following consensus statements pertaining to this topic. The results indicated:

- When the life care planner includes home care, both private-hire and agency-procured services are options to be considered.
- The cost of private-hire home care includes caregiver compensation and associated expenses.

Several points are worthy of further discussion:

- Care for the disabled child requires extraordinary physical and emotional commitment. The life care planner needs to assess the costs of assistive care as well as respite care when scheduling future needs.
- There may be a useful division in assistive care planning before and after 21 years of age. Up to age 21 years, care is most routinely provided by parents and schools. The individual need to care beyond basic parenting during these years should be clearly assessed. Thus, less assistive care may be needed before age 21 years.
- The type of long-term care is potentially a sensitive issue. The option of putting someone in a long-term skilled facility is generally less expensive, but advocates for the disabled argue that such facilities are an unsatisfactory setting to care for this population, and they should be reintegrated into the community.

How should care be delegated and priced? Different levels of care are provided by different nursing professionals: certified nursing assistants (CNA), licensed practical nurses (LPN, also known as licensed vocational nurses in some states), and RNs. Different states have differing Nursing Practice Acts defined by their legislature. The issue of delegation has become increasingly prevalent, and careful understanding for those who choose to delegate and those who do not wish to take on this responsibility (liability) should be evaluated and understood. The costs associated with hiring such professionals depend on their level of compensation. Although these rates may vary geographically, costs range from approximately $18 to $20/h for a CNA, $38/h for an LPN/LVN, and $56/h for an RN. The choice of professional is generally determined by the skilled nursing needs of the child. For example, are gastronomy tube feedings needed? Does the child require any type of drugs that are administered intravenously? Is the child partially or completely ventilator dependent? Does the delegation of care to less qualified caregivers put the patient at an unacceptable risk of injury or death? Is the child partially or completely ventilator dependent? These impairments alone may dictate the level of care required. In less physically compromised matters, appropriate foundation is required for using services beyond the obvious.

- Should the parents be expected to provide some of the care? The purpose of the life care plan is to promote independence in the least restrictive environment with consideration for safety and human dignity. In any setting, including litigation, the parents of a child with a diagnosis of cerebral palsy should undergo a clinical interview to consider the specifics of their individual family. Their ability to provide extraordinary care is likely determined by their health, number of other children, employment status, and other life roles.

- It may seem that private-hire care givers can be obtained for considerably less money than those obtained through nursing care agencies; however, associated expenses may alter this bottom line. Nursing care agencies prescreen, perform background checks, cover mandated state and federal employer costs, and ensure staffing needs are met. When hiring privately, an added burden may be placed on the family or they may not possess the capacity to perform the employer duties required to obtain and maintain quality care. The literature is mixed on this issue and provides no clear answer whether survival is better or worse with home versus institutional care.[8] The standards of practice speak to the need for thorough assessment of both options.

Future medical and surgical care

Rechecks with various specialties of physicians generally do not generate significant controversy within a life care plan. However, certain issues may arise:

- Should routine medical care be scheduled in a life care plan that would be required regardless of disability (eg, routine pediatric care, routine internal medicine care)? Transparency for routine needs and consideration given at the time of assessment and life care planning are appropriate.
- Items are included based on an appropriate foundation and their being medically reasonable, necessary, and appropriate. The life care planner develops recommendations for content of the life care plan cost projections for each client and a method for validating inclusion or exclusion of content.[30]
- Potentially controversial items include the need for a botulinum toxin, a baclofen pump for spasticity, or selective dorsal rhizotomy for spasticity, release of contractures, hip correction surgery for dysplasia, and scoliosis surgery. These subjects are dealt with each in turn.
- Botulinum toxin: the efficacy of botulinum toxin in treating spastic hypertonia in the child with cerebral palsy is beyond the scope of this review, and readers are referred elsewhere.[31] However, botulinum toxin is expensive (as much as several thousand dollars per treatment, with treatment effect lasting only 3 months), and the reduction of spasticity is not a goal in itself. Spasticity should be reduced when it interferes with care of the child, performance of activities of daily living, or gait.[32] A randomized trial showed no difference in a family's satisfaction with their child's function after botulinum toxin injection, despite improvement in both spasticity and function.[33]
- Baclofen pumps are another expensive option that should be considered only when they ease the patient's personal care or improve function. Baclofen pumps can cost as much as $15,000 when considering the charges of pump placement, pump replacement, programing and refilling, and the baclofen solution. Whereas oral baclofen is a generic drug, intrathecal baclofen is not. Again, readers are referred to other sources for comprehensive review.[31] However, evidence suggests that pumps reduce tone in children severely affected with cerebral palsy, but less so in ambulatory patients, and they are associated with considerable adverse affects.
- Selective dorsal rhizotomy surgery in patients with cerebral palsy has been debated for almost 25 years. Indications for the surgery are still not clear, and whereas some advocate the procedure in potentially ambulatory children with cerebral palsy, others advocate surgery for severely impaired children to ease perineal care.[31]

- Contracture surgery is a nonrecurring expense and does not add significantly to the total cost of a life care plan. It may be useful when it eases the care of a markedly contracted patient. Although it may provide benefits in the ambulatory patient, scores that measure gross motor function change little after surgery.[34]
- Hip dysplasia surgery is a nonrecurring expense and contributes minimally to the total cost of a life care plan. This surgery often alleviates the pain associated with the dislocated hip.
- Scoliosis surgery in the severely disabled child is highly controversial. Although neuromuscular scoliosis surgery may decrease the severe curve, evidence that it prolongs survival is not clear. Furthermore, in the severely impaired child, the ethical dilemma of whether to subject the child to an extremely painful, complication-prone, and costly procedure (approaching $100,000 when including surgical, anesthesiologic, and prolonged hospital stay for critical support) must be considered.[35]

Transportation and housing

When the child with a disability can no longer be lifted or transferred easily to a standard 4-door vehicle, transportation needs require attention. Key questions include the following: (1) is public transportation for the disabled person regularly available? and (2) should the entire cost of a wheelchair van be included in the life care plan, or only the modification costs? That is, if the typical cost of a wheelchair-accessible van is approximately $50,000, should the typical cost of a 4-door vehicle (approximately $26,000) be subtracted, leaving $24,000 as the cost included in the life care plan?

What adaptive housing costs should be included in a life care plan for a child with cerebral palsy? The Model Spinal Cord Injury Data Bank and the Veterans Administration provide useful figures for adaption of a home to wheelchair accessibility. Preliminary cost estimates based on the Department of Veterans Affairs allowance for veterans with service-connected disabilities are one-half the cost for modifications (up to a total of $63,780 allowed), to construct an adapted home or to modify an existing home.[36]

SUMMARY

This article synthesizes a large amount of information concerning life care planning in the child with cerebral palsy. Several key points summarize this review:

- A life care plan may be a useful construct to plan for and manage the needs of the disabled child with cerebral palsy.
- A cost analysis for a life care plan depends on the life expectancy of the child, and a careful review of the equipment, psychosocial, therapeutic, medical, nursing and domiciliary needs of the child.
- A wide variety of support services are available in the public sector, and it should be determined what services are reasonably available now and in the future.
- The lifespan of the child is curtailed by the presence of certain key disabilities, which are summarized in **Box 2**.
- Decreased cognitive abilities are associated with diminished life span, even in the absence of physical impairment.
- Life expectancy for physically and mentally disabled persons has increased slightly with time.
- No clear evidence suggests that institutionalized children have shorter life spans than those cared for in a noninstitutionalized setting.
- Advances in medical care have only slightly altered the poor prognosis for the most severely disabled children.

- The life care plan, whether completed by a physician or other qualified life care planner, must follow the generally accepted and peer-reviewed methodology with an appropriate foundation for each item recommended.

REFERENCES

1. Kuban KC, Leviton A. Cerebral palsy. N Engl J Med 1994;330:188–95.
2. Newacheck PW, Taylor WR. Childhood chronic illness: prevalence, severity and impact. Am J Public Health 1992;82(3):364–71.
3. Evans PM, Evans SJ, Alberman E. Cerebral palsy: why we must plan for survival. Arch Dis Child 1990;65:1329–33.
4. Rumeau-Rouquette C, Du Mazaubrun C, Mlika A, et al. Motor disability in children in three birth cohorts. Int J Epidemiol 1992;21(2):359–66.
5. Bush GW. Calculating the cost of long-term living: a four-step process. J Head Trauma Rehabil 1990;5(1):47–56.
6. Taylor JS. Neurolaw: towards a new medical jurisprudence. Brain Inj 1995;9: 745–51.
7. Katz RT. Life care planning for the child with cerebral palsy. J Missouri Bar 1996; 52:365–72.
8. Katz RT. Are children with cerebral palsy and developmental disability living longer? J Dev Phys Disabil 2009;21(5):409–24.
9. Eyman RK, Grossman HJ, Chaney RH, et al. Life expectancy of profoundly handicapped people with mental retardation. N Engl J Med 1990;323:584–9.
10. Life Expectancy for CP, VS, TBI and SCI. Correction of Eyman, et al. (1990) life expectancies. Available at: http://www.lifeexpectancy.com/eyman.shtml. Accessed August 19, 2012.
11. Shavelle RM, Straus DJ, Day SM. Comparison of survival in cerebral palsy between countries [letter to editor]. Dev Med Child Neurol 2001;43:574–6.
12. Plioplys AV, Kasnicka I, Lewis S, et al. Survival rates among children with severe neurologic disabilities. South Med J 2001;91:161–72.
13. Plioplys A. Deposition of Audrius Plioplys. Byron and Carolyn Simpson individually and as parents and next friends of Julia Simpson v. Texas Children's Hospital, Houston Pediatrics Surgeons et al. In: The District Court of Harrison County, Texas. June 20, 2006.
14. Singer LT, Kercsmar C, Legris G, et al. Developmental sequelae of long-term infant tracheostomy. Dev Med Child Neurol 1989;31:224–30.
15. Plioplys AV. Survival rates of children with severe neurologic disabilities: a review. Semin Pediatr Neurol 2003;10(2):120–9.
16. Strauss D, Shavelle R, Day S. Dr Audrius Plioplys' comparison of survival rates of children in the California data base and his own Chicago-area data base. Semin Pediatr Neurol 2004;11(3):236.
17. Strauss D, Shavelle R, Reynolds R, et al. Survival in cerebral palsy in the last 20 years: signs of improvement? Dev Med Child Neurol 2007;49:86–92.
18. Cohen A, Asor E, Tirosh E. Predictive factors of early mortality in children with developmental disabilities. J Child Neurol 2008;5:536–42.
19. Westbom L, Bergstrand L, Wagner P, et al. Survival at 19 years of age in a total population of children and young people with cerebral palsy. Dev Med Child Neurol 2011;53:808–14.
20. Reid SM, Carlin JB, Reddihough DS. Survival of individuals with cerebral palsy born in Victoria, Australia, between 1970 and 2004. Dev Med Child Neurol 2012;54(4):353–60.

21. Brooks JC, Shavelle RM, Strauss DJ. Survival in children with severe cerebral palsy: a further international comparison. Dev Med Child Neurol 2012;54:383–4.
22. Patja K, Iivanainen M, Vesala H, et al. Life expectancy of people with intellectual disability: a 35-year follow-up study. J Intellect Disabil Res 2000;44:591–9.
23. Bittles AH, Petterson BA, Sullivan SG, et al. Influence of intellectual disability on life expectancy. J Gerontol A Biol Sci Med Sci 2002;57(7):M470–2.
24. Tyrer F, Smith LK, McGrother CW. Mortality in adults with moderate to profound intellectual disability: a population-based study. J Intellect Disabil Res 2007;51: 520–7.
25. Tuel SM, Presty SK, Meythaler JM, et al. Functional improvement in severe head injury after readmission for rehabilitation. Brain Inj 1992;6:363–72.
26. Russman BS, Tilton A, Gormley ME. Cerebral palsy: a rational approach to a treatment protocol, and the role of botulinum toxin in treatment. Muscle Nerve 1997;6(93):S181–93.
27. Palmer FB, Shapiro BK, Wachtel RC, et al. Effects of physical therapy on cerebral palsy. A controlled trial in infants with spastic diplegia. N Engl J Med 1988; 318(13):803–8.
28. Olfson M, Marcus SC. National trends in outpatient psychotherapy. Am J Psychiatry 2010;167:1456–63.
29. Martelli MF, Zasler ND. Controversies in neuropsychology. NeuroRehabilitation 2001;16(4):195–7.
30. International Academy of Life Care Planners. Standards of practice for life care planners [review]. J Life Care Plan 2006;5(3):75–81.
31. Miller G. Management and prognosis of cerebral palsy. Available at: http://www.uptodate.com/contents/management-and-prognosis-of-cerebral-palsy. Accessed August 8, 2012.
32. Katz RT, De Wald J. Management of spasticity. In: Braddom RL, editor. Physical medicine and rehabilitation. New York: Saunders; 2000. p. 739–63.
33. Bjornson K, Hays R, Graubert C, et al. Botulinum toxin for spasticity in children with cerebral palsy: a comprehensive evaluation. Pediatrics 2007;120:49–58.
34. Abel MF, Damiano DL, Pannuzio M, et al. Muscle-tendon surgery in diplegic cerebral palsy: functional and mechanical changes. J Pediatr Orthop 1999;19: 366–75.
35. Phillips JH, Knapp DR, Herrera-Soto J. Mortality and morbidity in early onset scoliosis surgery. Spine (Phila Pa 1976) 2013;38(4):324–7.
36. United Stated Department of Veterans Affairs. VA announces amounts of assistance for veterans. Under the VA Specially Adapted Housing Program for fiscal year 2012. Available at: http://www.benefits.va.gov/homeloans/documents/docs/website_alert_2012.pdf. Accessed July 19, 2012.

Considerations for Neuropathic Pain Conditions in Life Care Planning

Judith P. Parker, MEd, CDMS, ABVE-D, CLCP[a],*,
Simone P. Javaher, RN, BSN, MPA[b], Frank K. Jackson IV, MS[c],
Gregory T. Carter, MD, MS[d]

KEYWORDS

- Neuropathic • Neuralgia • Peripheral • Autonomic • Psychogenic • Life care plan
- Chronic pain

KEY POINTS

- Neuropathic pain is a multifaceted phenomenon that can be difficult to alleviate.
- A life care plan, coordinated on behalf of a patient with neuropathic pain, requires many considerations, including the gender of the patient treated, the cause or causes of the neuropathic pain, and pharmacologic advances.
- Multiple modalities are available to be considered by a life care planner in conjunction with a physician.

INTRODUCTION

Pain is classified by duration (acute vs chronic) and pathophysiology (nociceptive vs neuropathic). Chronic neuropathic pain is caused by lesions in the peripheral or central nervous system (CNS) and can occur in many forms.[1–3] With neuropathic pain, nociceptive stimulation is not required, and the pain is disproportionate to the stimulation intensity. Pain signals are generated for unknown reasons and may be intensified if pain-relieving mechanisms are defective or deactivated.[4] Furthermore, a structure–function link between maladaptive dendritic spine plasticity and pain has been

Funding Sources: None to Disclose.
Conflict of Interest: None to Disclose.
[a] OSC Vocational Systems, Inc, Bothell, 10132 Northeast 185th Street, WA 98011, USA;
[b] Division of Pain Medicine, Department of Anesthesiology and Pain Medicine, University of Washington School of Medicine, 1959 Northeast Pacific Street, Box 356540, Seattle, WA 98195, USA; [c] Arizona College of Osteopathic Medicine, Midwestern University, Glendale, AZ 85308, USA; [d] Department of Clinical Neurosciences, Providence Medical Group, Olympia, WA 98506, USA
* Corresponding author.
E-mail address: judith@osc-voc.com

demonstrated previously in both CNS and peripheral nervous system injury models of neuropathic pain.[5]

Neuropathic pain is commonly seen in clinical practice and may be associated with a variety of peripheral nerve disorders, including neuropathy associated with diabetes, alcoholism, hypothyroidism, uremia, nutritional deficiencies, and chemotherapy, primarily treatment with vincristine, cisplatinum, zalcitabine, and paclitaxel. Other disorders that may be associated with neuropathic pain include almost all forms of hereditary and acquired neuromuscular disorders, including Charcot-Marie-Tooth disease; many forms of muscular dystrophy; Guillain-Barré Syndrome; postherpetic neuralgia; complex regional pain syndrome, type 1; and ischemic neuropathy.[6–23] Neuropathic pain afflicts an estimated 1.5% of the population worldwide.[24,25] In 2008, the analgesic market costs for neuropathic pain associated with diabetes alone were estimated at nearly $200 million annually and seemed to be rising.[26]

The range of therapeutic options to treat peripheral neuropathic pain has expanded greatly in recent years.[27–38] With proper treatment, most patients with neuropathic pain should experience a meaningful reduction in their pain and an improvement in quality of life.[39,40] A life care plan, coordinated on behalf of patients with neuropathic pain, requires many considerations. Life care planners look to the medical community to define the nature and extent of impairment. They use their specialized knowledge and clinical judgment along with established standards of practice.[41]

GENDER DIFFERENCES

Women and men perceive neuropathic pain differently and respond to treatment differently.[42,43] Women report more severe and longer-lasting neuropathic pain than men. Women and men also differ in their pharmacokinetic responses to treatments. Notable reasons for these differences include women having lower body weight and a higher percentage of body fat than men, which can affect the volume of distribution.[43] Adults are often given the same dose of drug regardless of body weight, so women tend to have higher serum concentrations of drugs than men receiving the same treatment. Other gender differences in bioavailability, metabolism, and renal elimination also may be involved in differing medication effects. In women, fluctuating body fluid mass during the menstrual cycle can affect drug blood levels, which changes glomerular filtration rates and subsequent renal drug clearance.

DIAGNOSIS

Pain involves an unpleasant physical sensation within the context of an individual's emotional, cognitive, and behavioral response to that sensation. Chronic neuropathic pain starts with pathophysiologic changes in the nerve, either from a medical condition (eg, diabetes) or direct trauma to the nerve (eg, a gunshot wound to brachial plexus), which leads to pain and inflammation. The injury heals but, if untreated, pain signals continue. Structural CNS changes alter neural transmission, resulting in chronic pain, hyperalgesia, allodynia, and occasionally the spread of pain. All of these symptoms should be considered when evaluating a patient with neuropathic pain. Despite the potentially complex cause, the diagnosis of neuropathic pain should be straightforward and is best made based on a patient's medical history and a physical examination. Ancillary testing, including electrodiagnostic testing, nerve imaging, or serologic studies, are not generally needed.[44] Small, unmyelinated C fibers may be involved in producing neuropathic pain, but these fibers are not assessed with traditional nerve conduction tests. Quantitative sensory testing may assess small fiber function using cold and cold/pain as well as hot and hot/pain detection threshold measurements.

In addition, quantitative sensory testing may provide information on abnormal sensory processing and perception.[45–47]

It is important to ask patients to describe their pain in detail, using descriptors rather than simply asking patients to rank pain intensity on a scale from 1 to 10. Patients suffering from neuropathic pain usually describe their pain as "electrical," "squeezing," "deep aching," "jabbing," "broken glass," "cramping," and "spasms." The Neuropathic Pain Scale (NPS), a validated assessment tool, is easily administered and provides an accurate characterization of neuropathic pain.[23] The NPS is easily accessed online[48] and lists 10 pain descriptors (intense, sharp, hot, dull, cold, sensitive, itchy, unpleasant, deep, and surface) that specifically describe common neuropathic pain qualities. The NPS provides clinicians with a reproducible appraisal of the degree and quality of neuropathic pain, which can be used to measure the efficacy of therapeutic interventions.

Allodynia and hyperalgesia are 2 critical physical examination findings in patients with neuropathic pain. Allodynia is pain caused by a normally nonpainful stimulus and can be assessed by simply stroking the skin lightly. Hyperalgesia is an exaggerated pain caused by a normally painful stimulus and can be assessed by a pinprick. With hyperalgesia, patients may initially say that they cannot feel a pinprick (sensory deficit), but after several pricks the sensation becomes quite painful. This phenomenon is known as summation. Moreover, the painful sensations may linger for seconds to minutes after the stimulus has stopped. This phenomenon is known as aftersensations. Pain described using the descriptors noted in the NPS along with the presence of summation and aftersensations are the critical elements that should be present in most patients with true neuropathic pain. Some patients with neuropathic pain, however, may not have allodynia or hyperalgesia.

MECHANISMS OF NEUROPATHIC PAIN

Neuropathic pain is caused by damage to the nervous system. Unlike physiologic pain, also known as nociceptive pain, neuropathic pain is not self-limiting. The causes of neuropathic pain are many and varied and include infectious agents, metabolic disease, neurodegenerative disease, and physical trauma, among other causes. Clinically, patients vary significantly in their response to treatment. The pathophysiology of neuropathic pain syndromes is complex. Many cellular mechanisms of pain transmission have been elucidated, and the clinical correlates of these mechanisms are beginning to be recognized. A variety of pathophysiologic processes may generate and maintain the symptom of pain in peripheral nervous system disorders. Conceptually, no one mechanism may be disease-specific, and each disorder may have several mechanisms typically associated with it. Thus, accounting for the pain in any individual patient may require hypothesizing that 1 or more mechanisms are at work simultaneously. For example, a patient with a drug-induced (toxic) neuropathy may share a pain mechanism with a patient who has a metabolic (diabetes) neuropathy. This heterogeneity may explain why only a subset of patients within each diagnostic category typically responds to a particular drug. Once neuropathic pain is present, all levels of the nervous system—peripheral, central, and autonomic—may play a role in generating and maintaining pain.[10] Therefore, independent of actual clinical diagnosis, several different pathophysiologic processes may be simultaneously present. Furthermore, some patients with neuropathic pain, especially those with mononeuropathies, may also develop secondary myofascial pain. It is imperative that clinicians realize that myofascial pain may mimic neuropathic pain and result in referred pain distant from the actual soft tissue source.[28]

Inflammation is thought to play a role as a pain generator in nerves. Eliav and colleagues[49] were able to induce an experimental neuritis in a rat by exposing the animal's sciatic nerves to an inflammatory stimulus. In this experiment, the investigators found statistically significant heat-hyperalgesia and mechano-hyperalgesia and mechano-allodynia and cold-allodynia in the inflamed nerve for 15 days, after which responses returned to normal. Light microscopic examination of the inflamed nerves, harvested at the time of peak symptom severity, revealed that the treated region was mildly edematous and that there was an obvious endoneurial infiltration of immune cells (ie, granulocytes and lymphocytes). There was either a complete absence of degeneration or degeneration of no more than a few 10s of axons. Immunocytochemical staining for CD4 and CD8 T-lymphocyte markers revealed that both cell types were present in the epineural and endoneurial compartments. The endoneurial T cells seemed to derive from the endoneurial vasculature rather than migrating across the nerve sheath. These results provide strong evidence that focal neural inflammation potentially produce neuropathic pain, even in the absence of significant or clinically detectable structural damage to the nerve.[49]

Furthermore, it is hypothesized and believed by most authorities that a primary neuropathic pain mechanism may be generated from ectopic impulses propagated from sites of abnormal or damaged nerve axons and the adjacent dorsal root ganglia.[50] Ectopic impulses are associated with a general increase in the level of neuronal excitability within primary afferent fibers and their synaptic contacts within the spinal cord. Novel, voltage-activated sodium channels are expressed at these sites and are thought to play an important role in generating ectopic impulses.[51] These channels are structurally diverse, comprised of several subunits, and may interact with extracellular matrix molecules to affect growth and myelination of axons. Differential regulation of the subunits by messenger RNA may contribute to the altered excitability of damaged neurons by influencing sodium channel function. Genetic influences may be present, because it has been shown that different strains of rats react differently to the same type of nerve injury. These differences may also been seen in the subsequently induced CNS changes.[51]

PHARMACOLOGIC MANAGEMENT

Despite much progress in pain research, neuropathic pain remains a formidable problem to manage. Many treatment options are available, yet less than half of patients experience clinically meaningful pain relief, which is almost always incomplete and significantly impairs their quality of life.[14] In addition, patients frequently experience adverse effects and, as a consequence, are often unable to tolerate treatment. In some patients, combination therapies using 2 or more analgesics with different mechanisms of action may provide adequate pain relief. Although combination treatment in clinical practice may result in greater pain relief, clinical trials with analgesic combinations are lacking. Trials with multiple drug combinations pose many methodological problems, including which combination to use, occurrence of additive or supra-additive effects, and the need for sequential or concurrent treatment. Adverse-event profiles of these analgesics are scarce, whether the analgesics are used alone or in combination. If pharmacologic pain management is ineffective, invasive therapies, such as intrathecal drug administration and neurosurgical stimulation techniques (eg, spinal cord stimulation, deep brain stimulation, and motor cortex stimulation), may be considered, although these treatments have not been well studied.

Even though many options are available to treat neuropathic pain, no clear consensus has been reached on which are most appropriate. Nonetheless, recommendations can be proposed for first-line, second-line, and third-line pharmacologic treatments based on the level of evidence available for different treatment strategies. Historically, most drugs used to treat neuropathic pain are considered adjuvant analgesics (ie, medications that are, by definition, agents whose primary indication is not analgesia). For example, tricyclic antidepressants (TCAs) and antiepileptic drugs (AEDs) have been mainstay treatments for neuropathic pain and include such pharmaceuticals as amitriptyline (Elavil) and gabapentin (Neurontin), a TCA and an AED, respectively.[52–56] Even today these drugs are used primarily as pain medications, although neither is approved by the Food and Drug Administration for this indication. Venlafaxine (Effexor) and other serotonin–norepinephrine reuptake inhibitors (SNRIs) may also be effective when used off-label to manage neuropathic pain, although limited data are available in humans to document their efficacy.[53,54] TCAs are often the first drugs selected to alleviate neuropathic pain (ie, they are a first-line pharmacologic treatment). Although they are effective in reducing pain in several neuropathic pain disorders, treatment benefit may be compromised and outweighed by their side effects.[55] Other options are needed in patients with a history of cardiovascular disorders, glaucoma, and urine retention. Newer drugs, for example, duloxetine (Cymbalta), also an SNRI, like venlafaxine, and pregabalin (Lyrica), an AED, may be better choices.[57–59] Unlike their predecessors, these drugs are FDA approved to treat pain. Pregabalin (Lyrica) also has documented efficacy in alleviating neuropathic pain and is now a first-line treatment for neuropathic pain.[58,59] Both pregabalin and gabapentin have more favorable safety profiles than older drugs, such as carbemazepine or phenytoin, with minimal concerns regarding drug interactions and showing no interference with hepatic enzymes.[60]

For refractory pain, opioids may alleviate nociceptive and neuropathic pain. The effectiveness of opioids in relieving acute pain has been well studied and established.[61,62] The use of opioids to treat any type of chronic pain, however, including neuropathic, remains controversial and is attributable in part to a lack of understanding of neuropathic pain and its mechanisms. Despite this contention, several randomized controlled clinical trials with opioids—morphine, oxycodone, and tramadol—were successful in helping alleviate neuropathic pain.[61] Tramadol is unique among opioids because of the additional serotonergic and noradrenergic signaling it stimulates.[62] Tapentadol (Nucynta), a newer drug, has both opioid and noradrenergic-stimulating components and is FDA approved for neuropathic pain.[62] Individual titration of opioid dosing and long-term follow-up studies are needed to measure long-term pain relief and to assess quality of life. Until that occurs, long-acting opioids, such as methadone, long-acting oxycodone (OxyContin), or morphine sulfate (MS-Contin), should be considered in patients whose pain is refractory to adjunctive agents.

Topical agents, including formulations of lidocaine, clonidine, capsaicin, and ketamine, are effective in treating localized neuropathic pain.[63–69] The efficacy of topical lidocaine patches (Lidoderm), and capsaicin ointment (Zostrix) is well documented in alleviating postherpetic neuralgia. Topical application is a novel approach to treating neuropathic pain and has the advantage of minimizing systemic side effects. If specific topicals are to be trialed for a patient, a compounding pharmacist can create customized formulations.

Recently included among these pharmacologic options is the use of cannabinoids, a class of drugs that take their name from *Cannabis sativa*, the botanic from which they were first isolated and which includes herbal preparations of cannabis as well as synthetic, semisynthetic, and extracted cannabinoid preparations.[70–72] Cannabis is administered mainly by 3 routes: via the lungs by inhalation of vaporized or smoked organic plant material; via the gut with ingestion of lipophilic, alcoholic, or supercritical fluidic extracts of plant material; or via the skin by topical application of plant extracts. Cannabinoids produce analgesia via supraspinal, spinal, and peripheral modes of action, acting on both ascending and descending pain pathways.[70] Cannabinoids are most commonly researched clinically for their role in managing neuropathic pain, but cannabinoids have also been used to treat malignant pain and other chronic pain syndromes, especially those involving hyperalgesia and allodynia, as well as acute pain applications.

COMPLEMENTARY AND ALTERNATIVE MEDICINE APPROACHES

Adding complementary and alternative therapies to conventional medicine may enhance treatment of neuropathic pain. To date, only preliminary data support combining alternative therapy with selected conventional medications for patients with neuropathic pain.[73-75] Randomized, controlled trials with appropriate control groups are needed to validate the effectiveness of this therapeutic approach. If Western medicine pharmacologic approaches are unsuccessful, however, then complementary and alternative medicine approaches, such as acupuncture, Chinese herbs, craniosacral therapy, and others, should be considered for individual patients as long as patients and clinicians are aware that the efficacy of this approach has not been systematically studied.

REHABILITATION MEDICINE APPROACHES

Patients with neuropathic pain may benefit from physical and occupational therapy modalities, including ultrasound, exercise, massage, orthotics, and bracing. A recent study showed that osteopathic manipulative treatment significantly alleviated chronic neuropathic pain associated with spinal cord injury over several weeks, coming remarkably close to the level of pain relief provided by standard pharmacotherapy.[76] At times, functional orthotics and bracing may also be helpful. A long-range management regimen should be oriented toward maximizing quality of life and minimizing comorbidity. For patients who have been deconditioned by immobility and lack flexibility, strength, or endurance, treatment often includes exercise.[77,78] Physical therapy encourages patients to use their own muscles to further increase flexibility and range of motion before advancing to other exercises that improve strength, balance, coordination, and endurance. To relieve pain, a physical therapist may use electrical stimulation, hot packs or cold compresses, ultrasound, traction, or deep tissue massage. Physical therapists may also teach patients to use assistive and adaptive devices, such as canes or braces, and instruct exercises for patients to do at home.

Occupational therapists help patients perform their activities of daily living independently and they may recommend using adaptive equipment to replace lost function.

Rehabilitation psychologists help patients relieve stress, cope with chronic neuropathic pain, and treat depression, all of which are common in patients suffering from chronic neuropathic pain.

IMPLANTABLE SYSTEMS FOR NEUROPATHIC PAIN—SPINAL CORD STIMULATORS AND PAIN PUMPS

When oral medications and/or nerve blocks do not sufficiently control neuropathic pain, advanced pain therapies or implantable systems may be effective treatments. These systems are designed to interrupt transmission of pain signals from the spinal cord to the brain so that patients do not actually feel the pain.[79-82] Spinal cord stimulation for pain control introduces low levels of electrical current to the dorsal portion of the spinal cord to block the sensation of pain. The device is surgically implanted, and may include a fully implanted system or one with an external power source.

Spinal pumps, also known as pain pumps, deliver pain-alleviating medication, typically morphine, directly to the intrathecal space around the spinal cord via an implanted pump. The pump is implanted surgically, and medication in the pump is added periodically (eg, monthly) by injecting medication through the skin into the pump reservoir. Spinal pumps may be used to manage chronic pain and spasticity. Multiple medications may be put into the pump to treat certain specific situations. For example, morphine may be used to treat nociceptive pain and local anesthetics can be added to treat a neuropathic pain component. For each of these procedures, a trial is first performed to see if it is effective and how patients respond before the surgery is performed. Both procedures are reversible and the implantable system can be removed.

LIFE CARE PLANNING FOR PATIENTS WITH NEUROPATHIC PAIN

Life care planning is governed by accepted standards of care, which include interprofessional specialty practice. As stated in an International Association of Rehabilitation Professionals International Academy of Life Care Planner standard of practice, "Each profession brings to the process of Life Care Planning practice standards which must be adhered to by the individual professional, and these standards remain applicable while the practitioner engages in Life Care Planning activities. Each professional works within specific standards of practice for his or her discipline to assure accountability, provide direction, and mandate responsibility for the standards for which they are accountable. These include, but are not limited to, activities related to quality of care, qualifications, collaboration, law, ethics, advocacy, resource use, and research."[41] Several consensus statements have been developed that guide life care planners. The many and diverse sources of neuropathic pain require coordination with a variety of medical specialists; however, the opinions of neurologists carry substantial weight with regards to future care needs.

Life care planning for chronic neuropathic pain requires an understanding of the complexities involved and the support of a skilled medical treatment provider. **Tables 1** and **2** show sample pages from an actual life care plan that has been coordinated with a neurologist. The tables demonstrate the various needs of a patient with neuropathic pain. Evaluation of patients includes a review of medical history, clinical observation, and a process of trial.[84] This helps identify future projected need for evaluations, medical care, and therapeutic modalities.

Adequate control of neuropathic pain is subject to a universe of treatments, each specific to patients. The hallmark of pain control, however, is medications. The National Guideline Clearinghouse is one resource for treatment guidelines for appropriate use of medications in these patients.[85] An understanding of the cause of the neuropathic pain, along with the expected progress of such pain, helps identify additional elements of the life care plan required over a patient's life expectancy. Examples include orthopedic needs, orthotic needs, home modifications, aids for independent functioning, durable medical equipment and supplies, wheelchairs, transportation needs, home care assistance, chore services, case management, and nursing care.

Appropriate nursing care options for different situations must be evaluated by a treating neurologist and may range from intermittent to constant care. The level of care depends on the degree of impairment and may be expected with a medical degree of certainty to progress over time. For example, peripheral neuropathies worsen over time and, should the precipitating factors remain unchanged, the condition is not

Table 1
Projected evaluations and future medical care

Item	Purpose	Provider	Age Initiated to Age Suspended	Replacement Rate	Base Cost[a]
Neurology	Evaluate neuropathic pain condition, recommend treatment	Current neurologist	Current age to life expectancy	Evaluation annually; follow-up 2–4 visits per year	
Neuro-ophthalmology	Evaluate vision status, recommend treatment as required	Neuro-ophthalmologist	Current age to life expectancy	Annually	
Pain management assessment and treatment	Pain management	Pain management physician	Current age to life expectancy	Annually; follow-up 2–4 visits per year	
Dietician	Monitor, evaluate and provide dietary guidance	Dietician	Current age to life expectancy	Evaluation twice; follow-up 1–2 times per month before total parenteral nutrition (TPN), (within 15 y), then daily monitoring until stabilized on tube feeding, then monthly	
Acupuncture	Evaluate for treatment of pain symptoms	Acupuncturist	Current age to life expectancy	Annually; follow-up twice weekly for the first 2 wk, then weekly	
Cognitive therapy	Speech/language therapies to promote executive functioning skills	Speech language therapist	Current age to life expectancy	Average annually	
Psychiatry	Medication management	Local psychiatrist	Current age to life expectancy	Average weekly	
Psychology	Treatment regarding psychological response to illness	Local psychologist	Current age to life expectancy	Average weekly	

[a] Base costs are typically included in the life care plan and should be nondiscounted/market rate prices from verifiable data from appropriately referenced sources that are geographically specific when appropriate and available, with more than one cost estimate, when appropriate.[83] "Accurate and timely cost information and specificity of service allocations that can be easily used by the client and interested parties" should also be identified.[41]

Table 2
Projected therapeutic modalities

Item	Purpose	Provider	Age Initiated to Age Suspended	Replacement Rate	Base Cost[a]
Acupuncture	Pain management secondary to neuropathic pain	Local provider	Current age to life expectancy	Twice weekly for the first 2 wk, then weekly	
Family counseling	Provide therapeutic setting for development of coping strategies	Local provider	Current age	Weekly for approximately 1 y	
Physical therapy	Provide strengthening and stretching to maintain balance, stability and range of motion	Local provider	Current age to life expectancy	Weekly 1-h sessions	
Occupational therapy	Provide coaching regarding maintaining activities of daily living	Local provider	Current age to life expectancy	Weekly 1-h sessions	
Massage therapy	Reduce pain, enhance mobility	Licensed massage therapist	Current age to life expectancy	2–4 Times per month	
Water therapy (Watsu)	Provide passive stretching therapy	Water massage therapist	Current age to life expectancy	1 h Weekly	

[a] Base costs are typically included in the life care plan and should be nondiscounted/market rate prices from verifiable data from appropriately referenced sources that are geographically specific when appropriate and available, with more than one cost estimate, when appropriate.[83] "Accurate and timely cost information and specificity of service allocations that can be easily used by the client and interested parties" should also be identified.[41]

expected to improve. These factors, spread over a remaining life expectancy, must be considered in life care planning. Escalating levels of nursing care can be expected in progressive conditions, such as multiple sclerosis, and the opinion of a treating neurologist determines the appropriate care specified in the life care plan.

In certain cases, an interprofessional pain management program may be appropriate. These programs include cognitive behavioral therapy, rehabilitation counseling, complementary and alternative medicine, interventional procedures, and other approaches that may provide optimal outcomes. In patients with complex pre-existing and unrelated addiction issues, treatment of pain that occurs after an injury is complicated. Health care providers must be careful to help patients comply with the pain management regimen without making ethical judgments of a prior condition. To protect patients, all parties must review the treatment plans closely, monitor protocols, track progress, and ensure that life care plans are current and relevant. Patients with less complex medical histories may also benefit from specialized pain programs. Here, treatment spans may be reduced and outpatient monitoring may be adequate for optimized outcomes. Life care plans may need to be monitored and updated regularly over time to maximize results and preserve quality of life.

SUMMARY

It is important for treating providers to understand the possible causes and mechanisms of neuropathic pain, the treatment options available, and the unique characteristics and circumstances of individual patients, to provide a regimen of care that maximizes quality of life. In concert with a neurologist and the interprofessional team, this level of knowledge and skill helps create and sustain an optimal patient-centered life care plan. The information included in a life care plan may require updating over time, depending on the age of a patient. Life care planners reflect these recommendations accurately and completely in a life care plan. Life care plans become the guide to future care.

REFERENCES

1. Jensen MP, Gammaitoni AR, Bolognese JA, et al. The pain quality response profile of pregabalin in the treatment of neuropathic pain. Clin J Pain 2012;28(8): 683–6.
2. Vranken JH. Mechanisms and treatment of neuropathic pain. Cent Nerv Syst Agents Med Chem 2009;9(1):71–8.
3. Calvo M, Dawes JM, Bennett DL. The role of the immune system in the generation of neuropathic pain. Lancet Neurol 2012;11(7):629–42.
4. Tan AM, Samad OA, Fischer TZ, et al. Maladaptive dendritic spine remodeling contributes to diabetic neuropathic pain. J Neurosci 2012;32(20):6795–807.
5. del Rey A, Apkarian AV, Martina M, et al. Chronic neuropathic pain-like behavior and brain-borne IL-1β. Ann N Y Acad Sci 2012;1262:101–7.
6. Engel JM, Kartin D, Carter GT, et al. Pain in youths with neuromuscular disease. Am J Hosp Palliat Care 2009;26(5):405–12.
7. Carter GT, Miro J, Abresch RT, et al. Disease burden in neuromuscular disease: the role of chronic pain. Phys Med Rehabil Clin N Am 2012;23(3):719–29.
8. Engel JM, Kartin D, Jaffe KM. Exploring chronic pain in youths with Duchenne Muscular Dystrophy: a model for pediatric neuromuscular disease. Phys Med Rehabil Clin N Am 2005;16(4):1113–24.
9. Galer BS. Painful polyneuropathy. Neuroimaging Clin N Am 1998;16(4):791–811.

10. Galer BS. Neuropathic pain of peripheral origin: advances in pharmacologic treatment. Neurology 1995;45(Suppl 9):S17–25.
11. Moulin DE, Hagen N, Feasby TE, et al. Pain in Guillain-Barre syndrome. Neurology 1997;48:328–31.
12. Suokas KI, Haanpää M, Kautiainen H, et al. Pain in patients with myotonic dystrophy type 2: a postal survey in Finland. Muscle Nerve 2012;45(1):70–4.
13. Carter GT, Jensen MP, Galer BS, et al. Neuropathic pain in Charcot Marie Tooth disease. Arch Phys Med Rehabil 1998;79:1560–4.
14. Abresch RT, Jensen MP, Carter GT. Health quality of life in peripheral neuropathy. Phys Med Rehabil Clin N Am 2001;12(2):461–72.
15. Abresch RT, Carter GT, Jensen MP, et al. Assessment of pain and health-related quality of life in slowly progressive neuromuscular disease. Am J Hosp Palliat Care 2002;19(1):39–48.
16. Jensen MP, Abresch RT, Carter GT. The reliability and validity of a self-reported version of the functional independence measure in persons with neuromuscular disease and chronic pain. Arch Phys Med Rehabil 2005;86(1):116–22.
17. Jensen MP, Abresch RT, Carter GT, et al. Chronic pain in persons with neuromuscular disorders. Arch Phys Med Rehabil 2005;86(6):1155–63.
18. Hoffman AJ, Jensen MP, Abresch RT, et al. Chronic pain in persons with neuromuscular disorders. Phys Med Rehabil Clin N Am 2005;16(4):1099–112.
19. Jensen MP, Hoffman AJ, Stoelb BL, et al. Chronic pain in persons with myotonic and facioscapulohumeral muscular dystrophy. Arch Phys Med Rehabil 2008; 89(2):320–8.
20. Molton I, Jensen MP, Ehde DM, et al. Coping with chronic pain among younger, middle-aged, and older adults living with neurologic injury and disease: a role for experiential wisdom. J Aging Health 2008;20:972–96.
21. Stoelb BL, Carter GT, Abresch RT, et al. Pain in persons with postpolio syndrome: frequency, intensity, and impact. Arch Phys Med Rehabil 2008;89(10):1933–40.
22. Carter GT, Jensen MP, Stoelb BL, et al. Chronic pain in persons with myotonic muscular dystrophy, type 1. Arch Phys Med Rehabil 2008;89(12):2382.
23. Miro J, Raichle KA, Carter GT, et al. Impact of biopsychosocial factors on chronic pain in persons with myotonic and facioscapulohumeral muscular dystrophy. Am J Hosp Palliat Care 2009;26(4):308–19.
24. Rodríguez MJ, García AJ. Investigators of Collaborative Study REC. A registry of the etiology and costs of neuropathic pain: results of the registry of etiologies and costs (REC) in neuropathic pain disorders study. Clin Drug Investig 2007; 27(11):771–82.
25. O'Connor AB. Neuropathic pain: quality-of-life impact, costs and cost effectiveness of therapy. Pharmacoeconomics 2009;27(2):95–112.
26. O'Connor AB, Noyes K, Holloway RG. A cost-utility comparison of four first-line medications in painful diabetic neuropathy. Pharmacoeconomics 2008;26(12): 1045–64.
27. Galer BS. Topical analgesic medication—the dawn of a new era. Pain 2009; 147(1–3):5–6.
28. Carter GT, Galer BS. Advances in the management of neuropathic pain. Phys Med Rehabil Clin N Am 2001;12(2):447–60.
29. Carter GT, Sullivan MD. Antidepressants in pain management. Curr Opin Investig Drugs 2002;3(3):454–8.
30. Backonja MM. Gabapentin monotherapy for the symptomatic treatment of painful neuropathy: a multicenter, double-blind, placebo-controlled trial in patients with diabetes mellitus. Epilepsia 1999;40(Suppl 6):S57–9 [discussion: S73–4].

31. Beydoun A. Postherpetic neuralgia: role of gabapentin and other treatment modalities. Epilepsia 1999;40(Suppl 6):S51–6 [discussion: S73–4].

32. Capsaicin Study Group. Effect of treatment with capsaicin on daily activities of patients with painful diabetic neuropathy. Diabetes Care 1992;15:159–65.

33. Chabal C, Russell LC, Burchiel KJ. The effect of intravenous lidoocaine, tocainide, and mexilitine on spontaneously active fibers originating in rat sciatic neuroma. Pain 1989;38:333–8.

34. Dejgard A, Petersen P, Kastrup J. Mexiletine for treatment of chronic diabetic neuropathy. Lancet 1988;2:9–11.

35. Galer BS, Harle J, Rowbotham MC. Response to intravenous lidocaine infusion predicts subsequent response to oral mexilitine: a prospective study. J Pain Symptom Manage 1996;12:161–7.

36. Max MB, Culname M, Schafer SC, et al. Amitriptyline relieves diabetic neuropathy pain in patients with normal depressed mood. Neurology 1987;7:589–96.

37. Max MB, Kishore-Kumar R, Schafer SC, et al. Efficacy of desipramine in painful diabetic neuropathy: a placebo-controlled trial. Pain 1991;45:3–9.

38. Max MB, Lynch SA, Muir J, et al. Effects of desipramine, amitriptyline, and fluoxetine on pain in diabetic neuropathy. N Engl J Med 1992;326:1250–8.

39. Von Korff M, Dunn KM. Chronic pain reconsidered. Pain 2008;138:267–76.

40. Tait RC, Chibnall JT, Margolis RB. Pain extent: relations with psychological state, pain severity, pain history, and disability. Pain 1990;41:295–301.

41. International Academy of Life Care Planners. Standards of practice for life care planners. J Life Care Plan 2006;5(3):75–81.

42. Werhagen L, Hultling C, Borg K. Pain, especially neuropathic pain, in adults with spina bifida, and its relation to age, neurological level, completeness, gender and hydrocephalus. J Rehabil Med 2010;42(4):374–6.

43. Werhagen L, Budh CN, Hultling C, et al. Neuropathic pain after traumatic spinal cord injury—relations to gender, spinal level, completeness, and age at the time of injury. Spinal Cord 2004;42(12):665–73.

44. Carter GT, Robinson LR, Chang VH, et al. Electrodiagnostic evaluation of traumatic nerve injuries. Hand Clin 2000;16(1):1–12.

45. Peripheral Neuropathy Association. Quantitative sensory testing: a consensus report from the peripheral neuropathy association. Neurology 1993;43: 1050–2.

46. Verdugo R, Ochoa JL. Quantitative somatosensory thermotest: a key method for functional evaluation of small caliber afferent channels. Brain 1992;15:893–913.

47. Mapi Research Trust. NPS (Neuropathic Pain Scale). Available at: http://www. mapi-trust.org/services/questionnairelicensing/catalog-questionnaires/74-nps. Accessed October 17, 2012.

48. Galer BS, Jensen MP. Development and preliminary validation of a pain measure specific to neuropathic pain: the neuropathic pain scale. Neurology 1997;48:332–8.

49. Eliav E, Herzberg U, Ruda MA, et al. Neuropathic pain from an experimental neuritis of the rat sciatic nerve. Pain 1999;83(2):169–82.

50. Amir R, Michaelis M, Devor M. Membrane potential oscillations in dorsal root ganglion neurons: role in normal electrogenesis and neuropathic pain. J Neurosci 1999;19(19):8589–96.

51. Devor M, Rappaport ZH. Pain and the pathophysiology of damaged nerve. In: Fields HL, editor. Pain syndromes in neurology. London: Butterworts; 1990. p. 47–85.

52. Watson CP, Vernich L, Chipman M, et al. Nortriptyline versus amitriptyline in postherpetic neuralgia: a randomized trial. Neurology 1998;51(4): 1166–71.

53. Lang E, Hord AH, Denson D. Venlafaxine hydrochloride (Effexor) relieves thermal hyperalgesia in rats with an experimental mononeuropathy. Pain 1996; 68(1):151–5.

54. Taylor K, Rowbotham MC. Venlafaxine hydrochloride and chronic pain. West J Med 1996;165:147–8.

55. McQuay HJ, Tramer M, Nye BA, et al. A systemic review of antidepressants in neuropathic pain. Pain 1996;68:217–27.

56. Morello CM, Leckband SG, Stoner CP, et al. Randomized double-blind study comparing the efficacy of gabapentin with amitriptyline on diabetic peripheral neuropathy pain. Arch Intern Med 1999;159(16):1931–7.

57. Cipriani A, Koesters M, Furukawa TA, et al. Duloxetine versus other anti-depressive agents for depression. Cochrane Database Syst Rev 2012;(10):CD006533. http://dx.doi.org/10.1002/14651858.CD006533.pub2.

58. Ogawa S, Satoh J, Arakawa A, et al. Pregabalin treatment for peripheral neuropathic pain: a review of safety data from randomized controlled trials conducted in Japan and in the west. Drug Saf 2012;35(10):793–806.

59. Semel D, Murphy TK, Zlateva G, et al. Evaluation of the safety and efficacy of pregabalin in older patients with neuropathic pain: results from a pooled analysis of 11 clinical studies. BMC Fam Pract 2010;11:85.

60. McQuay H, Carroll D, Jadad AR, et al. Anticonvulsant drugs for management of pain: a systemic review. BMJ 1995;311:1047–52.

61. Watson CP, Babul N. Efficacy of oxycodone in neuropathic pain: a randomized trial in postherpetic neuralgia. Neurology 1998;50(6):1837–41.

62. Raffa RB, Buschmann H, Christoph T, et al. Mechanistic and functional differentiation of tapentadol and tramadol. Expert Opin Pharmacother 2012;13(10): 1437–49.

63. Galer BS, Rowbotham MC, Perander J, et al. Topical lidocaine patch relieves postherpetic neuralgia more effectively than a vehicle patch: results of an enriched enrollment study. Pain 1999;80(3):533–8.

64. Rowbotham MC, Davies PS, Fields HI. Topical lidocaine gel relieves postherpetic neuralgia. Ann Neurol 1995;37:246–53.

65. Rowbotham MC, Davies PJ, Verkempinck CM, et al. Lidocaine patch: double-blind controlled study of a new treatment method for postherpetic neuralgia. Pain 1996;65:39–45.

66. Low PA, Oper-Gehrking TL, Dyck PJ, et al. Double-blind placebo-controlled study of the application of capsaicin cream in chronic distal painful polyneuropathy. Pain 1995;62:163–8.

67. Epstein JB, Grushka M, Le N. Topical clonidine for orofacial pain: a pilot study. J Orofac Pain 1997;11(4):346–52.

68. Fusco BM, Giacovazzo M. Peppers and pain. The promise of capsaicin. Drugs 1997;53(6):909–14.

69. Hardy J, Quinn S, Fazekas B, et al. Randomized, double-blind, placebo-controlled study to assess the efficacy and toxicity of subcutaneous ketamine in the management of cancer pain. J Clin Oncol 2012;30(29):3611–7.

70. Aggarwal SK, Carter GT, Sullivan MD, et al. Medicinal use of cannabis in the United States: historical perspectives, current trends, and future directions. J Opioid Manag 2009;5(3):153–68.

71. Aggarwal SK, Carter GT, Sullivan MD, et al. Characteristics of patients with chronic pain accessing treatment with medicinal cannabis in Washington State. J Opioid Manag 2009;5(5):257–86.

72. Carter GT, Flanagan A, Earleywine M, et al. Cannabis in palliative medicine: improving care and reducing opioid-related morbidity. Am J Hosp Palliat Care 2011;28(5):297–303.

73. Hui F, Boyle E, Vayda E, et al. A randomized controlled trial of a multifaceted integrated complementary-alternative therapy for chronic herpes zoster-related pain. Altern Med Rev 2012;17(1):57–68.

74. Hommer DH. Chinese scalp acupuncture relieves pain and restores function in complex regional pain syndrome. Mil Med 2012;177(10):1231–4.

75. Hsueh TP, Chiu HE. Traditional Chinese medicine speeds-up humerus fracture healing: two case reports. Complement Ther Med 2012;20(6):431–3.

76. Arienti C, Daccò S, Piccolo I, et al. Osteopathic manipulative treatment is effective on pain control associated to spinal cord injury. Spinal Cord 2011;49(4):515–9.

77. Löfgren M, Norrbrink C. "But I know what works"—patients' experience of spinal cord injury neuropathic pain management. Disabil Rehabil 2012;34(25):2139–47.

78. Simons LE, Kaczynski KJ, Conroy C, et al. Fear of pain in the context of intensive pain rehabilitation among children and adolescents with neuropathic pain: associations with treatment response. J Pain 2012;13(12):1151–61.

79. Sato KL, King EW, Johanek LM, et al. Spinal cord stimulation reduces hypersensitivity through activation of opioid receptors in a frequency-dependent manner. Eur J Pain 2012;12:43–7.

80. Meyerson BA, Linderoth B. Mechanisms of spinal cord stimulation in neuropathic pain. Neurol Res 2000;22(3):285–92.

81. Goto S, Taira T. Surgical procedures for neuropathic pain. Brain Nerve 2012;64(11):1307–13.

82. Nizard J, Raoul S, Nguyen JP, et al. Invasive stimulation therapies for the treatment of refractory pain. Discov Med 2012;14(77):237–46.

83. Preston K, Johnson C. Consensus and majority statements derived from Life Care Planning Summits held in 2000, 2002, 2004, 2006, 2008, 2010 and 2012. J Life Care Plan 2012;11(2):9–14.

84. Baron R, Förster M, Binder A. Subgrouping of patients with neuropathic pain according to pain-related sensory abnormalities: a first step to a stratified treatment approach. Lancet Neurol 2012;11(11):999–1005.

85. U.S. Department of Health & Human Services. National Guideline Clearinghouse. Available at: www.ngc.gov/. Accessed October 17, 2012.

Vocational Rehabilitation Process and Work Life

Rick Robinson, PhD, MBA, LMHC, CRC, CVE, CLCP, D/ABVE, NCC[a,b,*],
Sonia Paquette, OTD, OTR/L, CPE, ABVE-D[c,d,e,f]

KEYWORDS

- Vocational rehabilitation • Forensic rehabilitation • Work life • Work propensity
- Rehabilitation counseling • Labor supply • Labor demand • Earning capacity

KEY POINTS

- Private rehabilitation counselors use an established vocational rehabilitation process and work extensively in settings with the potential to be involved in legal proceedings.
- The vocational rehabilitation process and evaluation framework have given way to the vocational rehabilitation counselor's contemporary role as the generally accepted expert in vocational rehabilitation, evaluation, and vocational earning capacity assessment.
- To translate medical and functional information into life situation participation inhibitors or facilitators, the vocational rehabilitation counselor must know, understand, and take into account the contextual factors in which the injured person is most likely to exert those capacities.
- A person's ability to participate in the labor market can be complicated by disability-related issues, leading to a person experiencing periods of intermittent or decreased work availability over his or her remaining work life.
- Assessing impairment related to vocational functioning within a forensic context involves a complex and systematic review, evaluation, and synthesis of multiple domains of data that consider both the evaluee (labor supply) and the labor market (labor demand).

INTRODUCTION

The field of vocational rehabilitation grew out of a disability movement that has been developing and evolving over the past one hundred years. By the turn of the 20th

Funding Sources: None to disclose.
Conflict of Interest: None to disclose.
[a] Robinson Work Rehabilitation Services Co, PO Box 40050, Jacksonville, FL 32203, USA; [b] Department of Behavioral Science and Community Health, University of Florida, 1225 Center Drive, P.O. Box 100175 HSC, Gainesville, FL 32610, USA; [c] Ergonomics and Vocational Rehabilitation, Downingtown, PA 19335, USA; [d] Physical Therapy Post-Professional Doctorate Program, Rocky Mountain University of Health Professions, 561, East 1860 S, Provo, UT 84606, USA; [e] Occupational Therapy Transitional Post-Professional Doctorate Program, Rocky Mountain University of Health Professions, 561, East 1860 S, Provo, UT 84606, USA; [f] Master's and Doctorate Programs, Occupational Therapy, Salus University, 8360 Old York Road, Elkins Park, PA 19927, USA
* Corresponding author. Robinson Work Rehabilitation Services Co, PO Box 40050, Jacksonville, FL 32203.
E-mail address: rick@rwrehab.com

pmr.theclinics.com

century, the prevailing opinion toward occupational injuries was that "if the dangerous conditions were present when the worker took the job, he could be assumed to have accepted the risk and the possibility of injury [and] could not collect."[1(p13)] Workers' compensation laws were not part of the national conversation, as American business leaders feared that such laws would reduce profit margins by increasing business operating costs.[2] Despite these objections, the first compulsory state workers' compensation law was enacted in New York in 1910. By 1948, every state had adopted some form of workers' compensation legislation.[2]

Early workers' compensation laws did not explicitly provide vocational rehabilitation services, but such laws began to make legislators more aware of the need for vocational rehabilitation programs.[3,4] The first federal-state rehabilitation program (the Barden-LaFollette Act) was passed in 1948 and was intended to provide rehabilitation services to persons who were blind.[5] During World War II, significant medical advances were realized that further advanced the field of rehabilitation,[6] resulting in decreased rates of mortality for combat-related spinal cord injury, amputation, and burns.[6] Twenty years after the end of World War II, approximately 1400 of the 2500 soldiers experiencing combat-related paraplegia were employed.[7] With increased rates of survival came an increased need for long-term medical management of persons with chronic rehabilitative needs, leading to the American Medical Association beginning to view comprehensive rehabilitation management as the third phase of medical care, after the preventive and curative phases.[6] By 1947, the council that would ultimately become the American Board of Physical Medicine and Rehabilitation was charted by the American Medical Association.[6]

Between 1954 and 1965, funding for federal-state vocational rehabilitation services quadrupled to over $150 million.[4] The value of these services in 2012 dollars would be more than one billion dollars.[8] With increased federal funding also came increased costs for public-sector vocational rehabilitation efforts. In response, during the early 1970s, the insurance industry began to initiate private rehabilitation efforts aimed at cost containment and proactive rehabilitation initiatives.[9] Changing workers' compensation laws, greater public awareness of the cost of occupationally injured workers, and the general social attitude toward persons with disabilities helped give rise to a robust private vocational rehabilitation sector in the United States.[9]

From a practical perspective, private-sector and public-sector rehabilitation roles and goals are significantly different. Public-sector vocational rehabilitation efforts are typically more focused on assisting clients achieve maximum vocational potential.[10] Conversely, the primary focus of private-sector vocational rehabilitation typically revolves around returning an individual with a disability or injury to work, or establishing the potential of a person to work, earning compensation similar to what he or she was earning at the time of injury,[10] or in cases of diminished earning capacity, establishing the most probable earning capacity in work for which the individual retains vocational capacity. Private rehabilitation counselors use an established vocational rehabilitation process and work extensively in settings with the potential to be involved in legal proceedings.

VOCATIONAL REHABILITATION PROCESS

Rubin and Roessler described the vocational rehabilitation process as "a four-phase sequence, beginning with evaluation and moving through planning, treatment, and termination [placement]."[4(p289)] For any given case, the precise services provided by a vocational rehabilitation expert will depend on the context of the referral, funding source, regulatory requirements, and specific referral questions posed to the rehabilitation consultant. A vocational rehabilitation consultant may be involved in any one or all phases of the vocational rehabilitation process. For this article, emphasis is placed on the first 2 phases: evaluation and planning.

Nadolsky described vocational evaluation as a process intended to predict work behavior and vocational potential by applying vocational rehabilitation techniques and procedures.[11] Vocational evaluation is a process that systematically uses real or simulated work as the focal point for assessment and career exploration.[12] In conducting the evaluation, the vocational rehabilitation consultant synthesizes data from all rehabilitation team members that may include medical, psychological, economic, and other data sources such as cultural, social, and vocational information.

Since the genesis of vocational rehabilitation and evaluation, the research literature has contributed substantially to describing the factors and issues relevant to determining a person's vocational capacity. Assessment of disability related to vocational functioning involves evaluating multiple domains of both endogenous and exogenous variables. Individual, social, economic, and political influences merge to form the unique vocational and human capital profile an individual presents to an employer when being considered for work opportunity. Farnsworth and colleagues[13] wrote that the process of vocational evaluation draws on clinical skills from the fields of psychology, counseling, and education. Specific skills include file review, diagnostic interviewing, psychometric testing, clinical observation, data interpretation, and career counseling. These skills, when used within the vocational rehabilitation process, are important to evaluating a person's skills, abilities, and capacity to perform work activity for which the person is either qualified or may be able to become qualified.[14] The vocational rehabilitation process and evaluation framework have given way to the vocational rehabilitation counselor's contemporary role as the generally accepted expert in vocational rehabilitation, evaluation, and vocational earning capacity assessment.[14]

MEDICAL FOUNDATION FOR VOCATIONAL REHABILITATION ASSESSMENT

The ability of a person to perform the functions expected for occupational participation is predicated on the work capacity of that individual. The loss of a body function, a developmental delay, or an injury or illness may decrease a person's everyday functioning, including work functioning. Consequently, a medical condition leading to functional limitations or impairment may reduce a person's earning capacity. The ability to find a job, to sustain employment, or to attain higher levels of performance compared with a person with no impairment may lead to a vocational disability.

An important paradigm shift has occurred in the last 50 years in the construct of disability. Since the mid-20th century, disability was explained through the biomedical model,[15] where a linear relationship was assumed between the severity of a medical condition and the consequent severity of the patient's disability. The birth and increased popularity of Engel's biopsychosocial model in the late 1970s led to an important change in the perception and research approach toward disability. Disability is no longer seen solely as a medically related construct, but instead as an intricate melding of a variety of variables. These variables include not only the person's health condition but also the individual's activity restrictions, life situation participation, and contextual influences as inhibitors or facilitators of disability. The International Classification of Functioning[16] (ICF) framework was adopted in 2001 by resolution of the World Health Organization to explain and operationalize the interaction of health domains. The ICF considers functioning and disability as the 2 extremes in a continuum of health. A person's body functions and structures, previously seen in the biomedical model as the primary—if not unique—cause of disability, are now interacting with a person's activity participation or restrictions (the individual's level of capacity), as well as actual execution of those activities in his or her usual environment (the individual's level of performance). In this framework, disability is multidimensional. The medical condition is no longer the primary determinant of the disability's severity. The World Health Organization has operationally defined many of the key concepts for understanding the various constructs within the ICF paradigm[16]:

> *Body functions* are physiologic functions of body systems, including psychological functions.
> *Body structures* are anatomic parts of the body, such as organs, limbs, and their components.
> *Impairments* are problems in body function or structure, such as a significant deviation or loss.
> *Activity* is the execution of a task or action by an individual.
> *Participation* is involvement in a life situation.
> *Activity limitations* are difficulties an individual may have in executing activities.
> *Participation restrictions* are problems an individual may experience in life situations.
> *Environmental* factors comprise the physical, social, and attitudinal environment in which people live and conduct their lives.

In many countries, for legal and regulatory purposes, a causal relationship still needs to be generated to attribute responsibility for pecuniary damages, indemnity, and health-related service payments,[17] despite the knowledge that, even though a medical condition may have healed or not been diagnosed, the residual disability may linger because of other factors. As it is, medical and functional evidence constitute the necessary foundation to accept disability as a real entity. Therefore, a relationship must be established between the medical condition, the functional restrictions (ie, ICF's activity limitations), and the person's work disability (ie, ICF's participation restrictions).

Medical evidence is gathered by consulting with medical providers. Medical doctors are called on to establish disturbances in body structures and functions and to propose appropriate treatments to restore the body's premorbid health. Because of this knowledge and the lingering biomedical model still in effect in many policies and regulations regarding disability eligibility, medical doctors are often required or are expected to opine on work disability despite their lack of training, knowledge, and experience in diagnosing or treating disability as the ICF defines it.[18,19] Physicians specialized in disability rating are likely to rely on functional information to complement their medical findings and to define vocational readiness when such information is provided to them. Such information often comes from a functional capacity evaluation that is most typically (but not always) completed by an occupational or physical therapist.[20] For mental health disorders, psychiatrists, psychologists, and other licensed mental health professionals may provide diagnostic and treatment-related opinions. For people with brain diseases or injury, a neuropsychologist may determine the foci of structural and functional limitations.

This affects the forensic rehabilitation consultant in establishing the work-life participation and readiness. Under the ICF framework, the forensic vocational rehabilitation consultant is not able to extract life participation ("disability") information through simple activity restrictions provided by medical evidence because too many variables are missing. Medical and psychological evaluation findings are the result of a standardized or protocol-oriented approach that focuses on body structure and functions with a slight overlap on activity restrictions in a constrained environment. The ICF, as discussed earlier, defines this as capacity. However, work participation relates to performance within in a given context—where the environment changes, so too may performance, indicating that performance is seen as a separate entity from capacity, albeit most likely related, involving actual activity execution within a given environment.

To translate medical and functional information into life situation participation inhibitors or facilitators, the vocational rehabilitation consultant must know, understand, and take into account the contextual factors in which the person is most likely to exert those capacities. This complicates the picture, as the vocational rehabilitation consultant rarely has access to a potential environment in which the person could execute their capacities. However, knowing this margin of error helps the forensic vocational consultant present an opinion using a comfortable confidence interval, acknowledging those unobservable or untestable factors in the analysis and opinion formation. Through this personal and professional knowledge of the labor market, job demands, cultural and organizational demands of specific industries, and the current labor market, the vocational rehabilitation consultant may identify those missing criteria, exposing not only the gap in the predictive ability of the available determinants, but also explaining it. Only then can accurate work disability or readiness be established.

VOCATIONAL AND REHABILITATION ASSESSMENT

The opinions expressed by forensic vocational rehabilitation experts are typically presented as evidence in a legal venue and, as such, are subject to legal scrutiny under the rules of evidence for the venue in which the matter is being heard. The model for many rules of evidence is the Federal Rules of Evidence.[21] With respect to expert witness testimony, the Federal Rules of Evidence, Rule 702 reads:

If scientific, technical, or other specialized knowledge will assist the trier of fact to understand the evidence or to determine a fact in issue, a witness qualified as an expert by knowledge, skill, experience, training, or education, may testify thereto in the form of an opinion or otherwise, if (1) the testimony is based upon sufficient facts or data, (2) the testimony is the product of reliable principles and methods, and (3) the witness has applied the principles and methods reliably to the facts of the case.

Reliability of expert methods is of paramount importance if deference is to be given to an expert's opinions. According to Field and Choppa,[22] Rule 702 is important to vocational rehabilitation experts because it provides a basis for the admission of expert testimony on the grounds that vocational rehabilitation consultants possess unique knowledge, skill, experience, and training. Despite this, the vocational consultant must still demonstrate reliable application of methods and protocols in reaching conclusions. Barros-Bailey and Neulicht[23] proposed using both qualitative and quantitative data sources to describe how various factors interact and influence an individual's vocational characteristics. They referred to this hybrid method of integrating qualitative and quantitative data in rehabilitation case conceptualization as "opinion validity."[23(p34)] Moving from a purely quantitative approach to one that combines both quantitative and qualitative data analysis requires applying expert clinical judgment that is generally learned through one's training, skills, and experience. Choppa and colleagues[24] wrote about the need for one's clinical judgment to be predicated on an evidence-based scientific foundation as is practical. These authors described a model to apply clinical judgment that "incorporates such activities as direct observation, diagnosis (vocational evaluation and assessment), dispassionate (objective) and analytical observations, discerning and comparing (evaluating and synthesizing varieties of information), to assert a proposition (opinion) about the client."[24(p135)] The processes described by Barros-Bailey and Neulicht[23] and Choppa and colleagues[24] both illustrate the importance of integrating data from multiple sources to arrive at rehabilitation conclusions that are valid and reliable and would stand the test of legal scrutiny.

The Vocational and Rehabilitation Assessment Model (VRAM) (**Fig. 1**) is an empirically derived structural model of vocational and rehabilitation assessment specifically for use in forensic settings.[25] The structured presentation of VRAM is useful for visualizing the relationship and interaction of construct domains within the model. The model is divided into 3 distinct operational facets:

- Records review and rehabilitation interview (labor supply);
- Labor market research and inquiry (labor demand); and

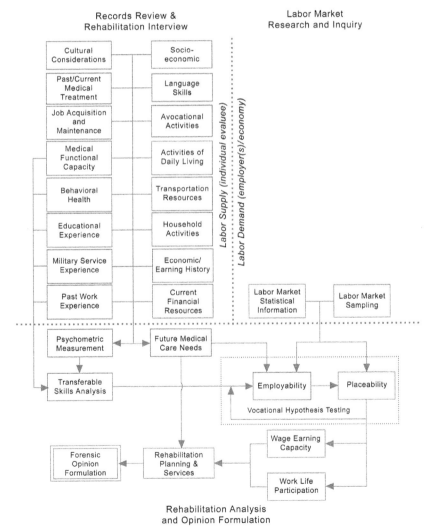

Fig. 1. Vocational and rehabilitation assessment model (VRAM).

- Rehabilitation analysis and opinion formulation, which represent the integration of the labor supply and labor demand aspects of the evaluation equation.

The balance of this article discusses each VRAM section and the data considered in each section.

RECORDS REVIEW AND REHABILITATION INTERVIEW

The records review and rehabilitation interview are, in most cases, requisite first steps in conducting a vocational and/or rehabilitation assessment. Conceptually, at this step in the assessment process, the rehabilitation consultant is focused on identifying the multitude of evaluee-specific variables expected to inhibit or facilitate present and future vocational and rehabilitation potential. Records review involves an analytical review of existing evidence with particular attention directed toward issues affecting vocational potential. Records review coupled with clinical interview findings are central to formulating a working hypothesis for further case-specific research, analysis, and vocational hypothesis testing. **Table 1** describes 16 core domains of data identified in a 2011 Delphi study.[26] These domains are considered essential elements in conducting a thorough vocational rehabilitation analysis. Not every data domain will necessarily apply in each case. However, to render the most accurate opinions possible, the vocational rehabilitation consultant has a responsibility to examine every element that may serve to influence the evaluee's vocational potential. Domains found not to be applicable after examination are simply left out of the equation, having gained the confidence that their exclusion will not influence the final analysis.

LABOR MARKET RESEARCH AND INQUIRY

Labor market information has long been an integral component in providing justification for vocational rehabilitation plans and opinions.[27,28] In fact, Gilbride and Burr believed labor market information to be as important to the vocational evaluation process as information about the evaluee himself.[28] Labor market research and inquiry involve analyzing and synthesizing multiple data sources to test hypotheses related to an evaluee's vocational employability and placeability.[25] The focus of inquiry may center on any number of data sources, such as government, proprietary, or trade industry employment and wage statistics, employment projections, studies of occupational density, and labor market surveys. The principal focus of labor market research and inquiry should be synthesis of multiple data sources to ultimately arrive at a conclusion of an evaluee's vocational potential.

Although large sample statistical sources may provide insight into an array of vocational and employment issues, often they do little to provide insight into local labor market conditions. Many governmental surveys, studies, and large sample databases are intended for econometric application to make broad generalizations on national or regional policy trends, not conclusions about how the data may apply to a single individual.[29] For forensic vocational rehabilitation, the labor market survey demonstrates the availability, wage characteristics, and other relevant data for specific occupations, during a specific period of time, and within a specific geographic scope.[30] Barros-Bailey defined the labor market survey as a "survey methods strategy to collect qualitative and/or quantitative data for a small population census or sample about an identified labor market to draw inferences to the client/evaluee (N = 1)."[27(p137)] The labor market survey provides ecological validity to expert opinions of vocational capacity.

Barros-Bailey described the labor market survey as a "means of ergometric and ergonometric data collection that could help bridge information with econometric

Table 1
Record review and clinical interview domains

Domain	Operational Definition	Clinical Interview	Review of Existing Records	Observation	Psychometric Measurement	Provider Consultation
				Typical Data Source		
Activities of daily living	Variables addressing self-care issues and assistance received either through personal care services or assistive devices and equipment	✓	✓			
Avocational activities	Variables related to hobbies and recreational pursuits	✓	✓			
Behavioral health	Variables that describe the behavioral relationship between the individual and his or her immediate and extended social environments	✓	✓	✓	✓	✓
Cultural considerations	Variables that describe the behaviors and beliefs characteristic of a particular social, ethnic, or other group	✓		✓		
Current financial resources	Variables that address the financial health, status, and stability of the evaluee	✓	✓			
Economic and earning history	Variables that address a person's current and historical personal income and resources	✓	✓			

Variable	Description			
Educational experience	Variables that address a person's primary, secondary, vocational, and apprentice educational development	✓		
Household activities	Variables that address the evaluee's participation in household activities	✓		
Job acquisition and maintenance	Variables that address issues related to obtaining and maintaining work	✓		
Language skills	Language skills variables that address language skills	✓	✓	
Medical functional capacity	Variables that address a person's residual functional capacity for activity and function	✓		✓
Military service experience	Variables related to a person's military service experience	✓		
Past and current medical treatment	Variables related to a person's past medical history and current medical treatment	✓		
Past work experience	Variables specific to each individual job held over a person's work history	✓		
Socioeconomic	Variables that address individual, social, and economic factors that are specific to the evaluee	✓		
Transportation resources	Variables that address transportation-related skills and barriers	✓		

data sources to client/evaluee needs."[27(p7)] In other words, large-sample econometric data sources such as governmental statistics and survey data, in concert with local labor market survey data that are highly focused on a very specific geography, occupation, and personalized vocational profile, merge to provide the clearest possible picture of vocational capacity and potential.

REHABILITATION ANALYSIS AND OPINION FORMULATION

Rehabilitation analysis and opinion formulation involve application of established vocational rehabilitation methods and protocols that, along with the other VRAM sections, contribute to developing expert vocational and rehabilitation opinions. Because of the varying nature and venue of cases, the specific analyses performed require professional judgment to address necessary referral questions. Core vocational and rehabilitation analyses may include any or all of the following:

- Psychometric measurement
- Analysis of future medical care needs
- Transferable skills analysis
- Analysis of employability
- Analysis of placeability
- Analysis of earning capacity
- Analysis of work-life participation

PSYCHOMETRIC MEASUREMENT

Psychometric measurement of various worker traits provides key data for analyzing rehabilitation need and employment potential. Psychometric assessment instruments are evaluee specific and require professional judgment to ensure appropriate instrument selection. The most common instruments administered at this stage include measures of intelligence, educational achievement, aptitudes, interests, personality, and temperament. Data stemming from psychometric assessment are key to developing a residual vocational and rehabilitation profile for subsequently analyzing transferable skills to other work.

FUTURE MEDICAL CARE NEEDS

Generally speaking, the more intensive future medical care needs are, the greater the impact on a person's ability to sustain and maintain competitive employment.[31,32] The need for future medical care related to a chronic health care condition not only can affect future vocational participation but also is integral to describing the future health needs in cases where the rehabilitation consultant is retained to complete a life care plan. Apart from development of a life care plan, the time requirements, frequency, and duration required to participate in future medical care can have a direct impact on both formulation of a rehabilitation plan and an evaluee's vocational potential.

TRANSFERABLE SKILLS ANALYSIS

Power described the following 3 types of skills: adaptive, functional, and content skills.[33] Adaptive skills are related to individual self-management and personality traits. Functional skills are individual behaviors or abilities related to interaction with data, people, and things within a work environment or context. Content skills are best described as competencies a person has that are directly related to performance of a specific job or cluster of jobs. In cases where an evaluee cannot return to his or her previous work because of reduced functional capacity, it is necessary to identify suitable jobs within the person's functional skill level. If applicable, identifying an evaluee's preinjury skills is a requisite step to identifying alternative vocational opportunities or jobs.

EMPLOYABILITY AND PLACEABILITY

The concepts of vocational employability and placeability are core elements in nearly every assessment of vocational capacity. Employability addresses whether an evaluee is ready for work. Central employability issues involve selection of appropriate vocational goals that consider the evaluee's vocational readiness characteristics, such as aptitudes, personality, temperament, and residual functional capacity. Although employability addresses work readiness issues, placeability addresses whether an individual meets the hiring requirements of actual employers within a specific geographic labor market. Although a job may exist within a particular labor market, if the evaluee in question is not a reasonable candidate for employment consideration, then the suitability of the job as a vocational goal must be questioned. To be considered a viable work opportunity, the concepts of vocational employability and placeability must be demonstrated jointly.

WAGE EARNING CAPACITY

In many litigated settings, the end result of litigation is a determination of the injuries or damages sustained by a claimant or plaintiff.[34] Often, economic damages caused by a loss or reduction in a person's ability to earn wages or a salary can be significant and represent a large proportion of the total damages sought to be recovered.[35] In many venues, damages from lost wages because of an injury or death are measured by an earning capacity standard, rather than an actual or expected earnings standard.[36] An actual earning standard would only acknowledge the historical earning record of a person and would not be prospective. According to Horner and Slesnick, actual earnings are best conceptualized as a "series of outcomes of a complex stochastic process involving the interaction of a person's abilities and preferences with the needs of employers."[36(p14)] An expected earnings standard is simply "a series of earning figures, which are the expected values of actual earnings in the corresponding time periods."[36(p14)] Expected earnings rely on a more mathematical solution and therefore are not directly observable. Because of the mathematical foundation of an expected earnings standard, it does not account for changes in future earnings influenced by the unique vocational factors of the individual—namely, the individual's abilities, available work opportunities, and the individual's vocational orientation toward future work. Simple reliance on a person's past vocational decisions to project a future vocational course can be flawed, particularly in cases involving injury or a reduction in functional capacity for future work.

Using an earning capacity standard, the expert's opinions will consider the expected earnings of a worker who chooses to maximize actual earnings. Accordingly, earning capacity is not normally affected by voluntary vocational choices made by a worker regardless of whether the choice is made to exercise inherent abilities or not. Earning capacity opinion formulation is highly complex and involves synthesizing the multitude of data elements considered in the assessment model.

WORK-LIFE PARTICIPATION

When evaluating losses related to a reduction in a worker's prospective vocational capacity, it is often necessary to estimate the number of years over which the loss is likely to occur. This estimate is referred to as a worker's work-life expectancy. Alter and Becker stated a person's work life "is then used to calculate the present value of expected earnings lost between the date of death or injury and the date of expected final separation from the work force."[37(p39)] On the surface, this estimate may seem to be a straightforward process that is easily calculated. In reality, estimating a person's work-life expectancy is an imperfect process that is far from straightforward. Unlike estimating a person's life expectancy, which is measured by 2 discrete events—birth and death—a person's work behavior is not so clear and may change over time. Because a person's work behavior is not static, determining whether a person is working, is looking for work, or is only marginally attached to the labor market is not clearly defined or easily measured. For example, a worker may

- Hold multiple jobs or work significant amounts of overtime[38];
- Work unpaid in a family-owned business[39,40];
- Voluntarily or involuntarily limit participation to part-time work for economic or noneconomic reasons[41];
- Experience changing family roles resulting in constrained choice[42]; and
- Be marginally attached to the labor force because of futility of job search efforts or discouragement.[38]

A person's participation in the labor force is even less clear when disability is involved. Disability may interact or interfere with the person's ongoing participation in the labor market, causing periods of interruption or inactivity. A 2009 Bureau of Labor Statistics report shows a strong relationship between disability and discontinuous or decreased participation in the labor force.[43] Highlights from this report indicate

- For all ages, the employment-population ratio was much lower for persons with a disability than for those with no disability;
- The unemployment rate of persons with a disability was well above the rate of those with no disability;
- Persons with a disability were over 3 times as likely as those with no disability to be age 65 or over; and
- Nearly one-third of workers with a disability were employed part time, compared with about one-fifth of those with no disability.[43(p1)]

A person's ability to participate in the labor market can be complicated by disability-related issues. These issues may lead a person to experience periods of intermittent or decreased work availability over his or her remaining work life. Disability may temper or moderate a worker's ability to participate in the labor market full time or to full retirement age. As an example, a person may be medically limited to part-time work of 4 hours per day, while their historical participation was 8 hours per day. Here, the employee continues to participate in the labor market, albeit at only 50% of his or her predisability participation rate, thus resulting in a 50% reduction in work availability for his or her remaining work life. The interaction of disability and work capacity is even less clear in cases where a worker continues to work full time but is projected to reduce work participation either intermittently or prospectively over his or her remaining work life.

The concept of work-life expectancy has been variously defined by authors over the past several decades. Foster and Skoog define work life as "the duration of time a person will spend either working or actively looking for work during the remainder of his or her life."[44(p167)] This definition focuses principally on the activity of work or job search as the foundation for a person's work-life expectancy. Gamboa and Gibson defined work life as the "total number of years in aggregate that an individual is likely to be alive and employed."[45(p7)] This definition focuses attention more on the act of working to the exclusion of the amount of time a person may not be employed, yet may be participating in the labor market through job search efforts. Even though job search efforts do not affect immediate earnings quantitatively, they may very well influence future earnings. Ireland defined work-life expectancy as "the number of years and partial years that a worker would be expected to participate in the labor market before either death or final retirement from the labor market."[46(p112)] Ireland's definition includes consideration of full-time and part-time employment as well as participation, which may include periods during which a worker is unemployed, yet actively looking for work.

Estimating a person's work-life expectancy is similar in process to evaluating a person's loss of earning capacity. When evaluating a person's loss of earning capacity after impairment, the rehabilitation consultant must first have a reasonable understanding of the evaluee's preimpairment earning capacity. The preimpairment capacity is then compared with the evaluee's postimpairment earning capacity to determine the degree of loss. Similarly, when estimating a person's work-life expectancy, the forensic rehabilitation consultant must first have a reasonable understanding of how long the person was likely to have remained in the labor market were it not for the intervening impairment. Multiple statistical models of work-life expectancy have been published for estimating a person's nonimpaired work life.[47–49]

According to Field and Jayne, when using statistical work-life expectancy tables, it "may be more appropriate to consider disability issues through a process of clinical judgment, including a proper assessment, based on a medical foundation, of the individual's functional capacities and the impact the disability (probable reduced functioning) will have on the person's ability to work and earn money."[50(p83)] Robinson and Spruance described these disability and related adjustments to an evaluee's statistical work-life expectancy estimate as work propensity theory.[51] Future work propensity factors may moderate a person's propensity for future participation in the labor market cumulatively, intermittently, or terminally. Instead of estimating a person's future work participation based solely on statistical models, work propensity theory uses both qualitative and quantitative data to present a "range of reality" with respect to the evaluee's postimpairment work-life expectancy.[51(p31)] Considering both qualitative and quantitative data sources together allows the forensic rehabilitation consultant to describe how work propensity factors may interact and/or influence the individual. In the absence of individualized work-life estimates, the forensic rehabilitation consultant is left to rely solely on large-sample homogenized statistical estimates that may not be at all representative of the unique characteristics of the person being evaluated. Accordingly, work propensity factors are best viewed as a practical educative adjunct to purely statistical approaches to work-life expectancy that may be more easily understood by a jury or trier of fact.

Assessment of work propensity factors is not a cookbook method of statistics but instead requires applying expert clinical judgment and interpretation of the many factors that may influence the interaction between the worker (labor supply) and the employer/labor market (labor demand) in the future. The interaction between economic supply and demand factors will determine market conditions under which workers are hired, retained, and promoted. Within an economic supply-and-demand model, the market will define the necessary skill set for a worker to obtain jobs in his or her chosen profession. Supply-side factors are presented to an employer by an employee being considered for employment, which include variables such as an individual's functional capacity, vocational capacity, and worker preferences.[36] Demand-side factors are external to the individual being evaluated and are a function of the number of jobs available with employers at a given wage rate and for a specific vocational capacity profile.[36] Demand-side factors include considerations such as local demographics and geography for a particular labor market, the unemployment rate, and the availability or supply of workers matching the necessary vocational profile. Within an ideal free market economy, competitive employment results when a fit is realized between the demand for a certain vocational profile (employer) and the supply of the needed labor (employee). It is the interaction of these 2 economic forces upon the 12 work propensity domains that theoretically will determine the duration of time a person will remain active and actively participating in the labor market (**Fig. 2**).

REHABILITATION PLANNING AND SERVICES

Rehabilitation planning involves developing and detailing an evaluee-specific plan aimed at sustaining or improving physical, psychosocial, educational, and vocational functioning. Developing the rehabilitation plan involves considering data extracted throughout the VRAM model. Data are synthesized into recommendations that, where practical, are operationalized into measurable objectives with a specific timeline and, when possible, associated costs.

OPINION FORMULATION

Opinion formulation involves summarizing the many conclusions that are drawn throughout the assessment model. For example, the basic foundation of variables is identified through file review and a clinical interview. Conclusions drawn from review of records and the interview provide the foundation for psychometric instrument selection, transferable skills analysis, and clarification of future medical care needs. These findings directly influence the employability and placeability analysis of jobs considered suitable for the evaluee. Once conclusions are drawn regarding an evaluee's vocational employability and placeability, opinions are then formed of the evaluee's earning capacity and work-life participation. Each conclusion drawn to this point influences and guides the formulation of the rehabilitation plan and service

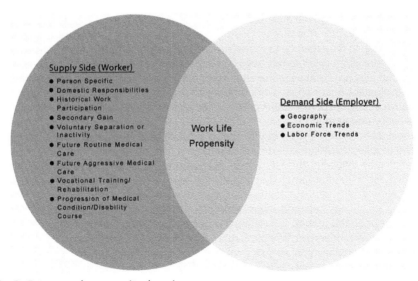

Fig. 2. Future work propensity domains.

recommendations for the evaluee. Each decision or conclusion drawn should be summarized, as this allows opinions and conclusions to be clearly stated. Such a summary may also be useful for presenting opinions and conclusions to a trier of fact or jury.

SUMMARY

Assessing impairment as it relates to vocational functioning within a forensic context involves the systematic review, evaluation, and synthesis of multiple domains of data. Individual, social, political, economic, and health-related factors merge to form the unique vocational profile an individual presents to the labor market when being considered for work opportunity. The foundation of the assessment must rest on a solid medical foundation that clearly describes the evaluee's impairment and quantifies the work capacity of the evaluee. Only after the work capacity is established may the vocational rehabilitation consultant embark on the vocational assessment process and determine if the impairment is likely to result in a vocational disability. It is necessary to understand that the concept of disability should not be viewed from a medical perspective alone, but instead from a multifaceted perspective that considers the health condition, body functions and structures, activities, participation, and environmental and personal factors.

To evaluate the presence, pervasiveness, and scope of a vocational disability, it is necessary to evaluate the core domains of vocational function. An empirically sound model for conducting such an assessment is the VRAM, a 3-facet assessment model that includes a review of records and rehabilitation interview (labor supply); labor market research and inquiry (labor demand); and rehabilitation analysis and opinion formulation, which integrate the labor supply and labor demand aspects to the model.

Within the rehabilitation analysis and opinion formulation facet of VRAM is the need to estimate the evaluee's work-life expectancy. Work-life expectancy results from a nonlinear process involving a wide variety of variables specific to the person and his or her environment. A common method to establish work-life expectancy is to use one or more of the published statistical tables. Although this method may provide a statistic that is offered as a reasonable proxy of the person's work-life expectancy, it is important not to simply apply the person to the statistic. The authors of this article contend that because of the importance that work-life expectancy plays in calculating total loss estimates, the length of an individual's work life is too important to be so arbitrarily established without adjustments that consider the unique characteristics of the evaluee. Work-life expectancy estimates should be adjusted to reflect the supply and demand variables likely to influence the amount of time the evaluee may remain in the labor market. In composite, evaluating an individual's future vocational capacity and work-life expectancy involves a multifaceted and complex examination of a range of variables. Because the evaluation is conducted within a forensic setting, the rules of evidence must be considered for the jurisdiction in which the matter is being heard. Accordingly, consistent and reliable application of the assessment model is crucial to ensure the legal admissibility of vocational expert opinions and conclusions to a jury or trier of fact.

REFERENCES

1. Obermann CE. The limitations of history. In: Wright GN, editor. Madison lectures on vocational rehabilitation. Madison (WI): The University of Wisconsin, Rehabilitation Counselor Education Program; 1967.

2. Safilios-Rothschild C. The sociology and social psychology of disability and rehabilitation. New York: Random House; 1970.
3. Obermann C. A history of vocational rehabilitation in America. Minneapolis (MN): TS Dennison & Company; 1965.
4. Rubin SE, Roessler RT. Foundations of the vocational rehabilitation process. 6th edition. Austin (TX): Pro-Ed; 2008.
5. Switzer M. Legislative contributions. In: Malikin D, Rusalem H, editors. Vocational rehabilitation of the disabled: an overview. New York: University Press; 1969. p. 39–53.
6. Allan WS. Rehabilitation: a community challenge. New York: Wiley; 1958.
7. Rusk H. A world to care for. Pleasantville (NY): Reader's Digest Condensed Books; 1972.
8. U.S. Department of Education. Remarks of U.S. Secretary of Education Arne Duncan to the SHEEO Higher Education Policy Conference. Available at: www.ed.gov/news/speeches/remarks-us-secretary-education-arne-duncan-sheeo-higher-education-policy-conference. Accessed September 7, 2012.
9. Weed R, Field T. Rehabilitation consultant's handbook. Revised edition. Athens (GA): Elliott & Fitzpatrick; 2001.
10. Rasch J. Rehabilitation of workers compensation and other insurance claimants. Springfield (IL): Charles C. Thomas; 1985.
11. Nadolsky J. Vocational evaluation theory in perspective. Rehabil Lit 1971;32(8): 32–8.
12. Vocational Evaluation and Career Assessment Professionals (VECAP). Three levels of vocational assessment. Available at: www.vecap.org/images/uploads/docs/Levels_of_Assessment.pdf. Accessed September 15, 2010.
13. Farnsworth K, Field J, Field T, et al, editors. The quick desk reference for forensic rehabilitation consultants. Athens (GA): Elliott & Fitzpatrick; 2005.
14. Owings S, Lewis S, Streby C, et al. A rehabilitation counselor's practical and historical guide to earning capacity assessment. Athens (GA): Elliott & Fitzpatrick; 2007.
15. Engel GL. The need for a new medical model: a challenge for biomedicine. Science 1977;196:129–35.
16. World Health Organization. International classification of functioning, disability and health. Geneva (Switzerland): Author; 2001.
17. Anner J, Schwegler U, Kunz R, et al. Evaluation of work disability and the international classification of functioning: what to expect and what not. BMC Public Health 2012;12:470.
18. Denez Z, Fazekas G, Zsiga K, et al. Physicians' and medical students' knowledge on rehabilitation. Orv Hetil 2012;24:954–61 [in Hungarian].
19. Soklaridis S, Tang G, Cartmill C, et al. "Can you go back to work?" Family physicians' experiences with assessing patients' functional ability to return to work. Can Fam Physician 2011;57:202–9.
20. Wind H, Gouttebarje V, Kuijer PP, et al. Complementary value of functional capacity evaluation for physicians in addressing the physical work ability of workers with musculoskeletal disorders. Arch Occup Environ Health 2009; 82(4):435–43.
21. U.S. House of Representatives. Federal rules of evidence. Washington, DC: Committee on the Judiciary; 2009.
22. Field TF, Choppa AJ. Admissible testimony: a content analysis of selected cases involving vocational experts with a revised clinical model for developing opinion. Athens (GA): Elliott & Fitzpatrick; 2005.

23. Barros-Bailey M, Neulicht A. Opinion validity: an integration of quantitative and qualitative data. The Rehabilitation Professional 2005;13(2):33–41.
24. Choppa A, Johnson C, Fountain J, et al. The efficacy of professional clinical judgment: Developing expert testimony in cases involving vocational rehabilitation and care planning issues. J Life Care Plan 2004;3(3):131–50.
25. Robinson R, Pomeranz J. The vocational and rehabilitation assessment model (VRAM): introduction of an empirically derived model of forensic vocational and rehabilitation assessment. The Rehabilitation Professional 2011;19(4):91–104.
26. Robinson R. Identification of core variables to be considered in an assessment of vocational earning capacity in a legal forensic setting: a Delphi study. Doctoral dissertation. 2011. Available at: http://etd.fcla.edu/UF/UFE0043197/robinson_r.pdf. Accssed November 10, 2012.
27. Barros-Bailey M. Commentary: labor market survey methodology and applications. The Rehabilitation Professional 2012;20(2):137–46.
28. Gilbride D, Burr F. Self directed labor market survey: an empowering approach. Journal of Job Placement 1993;9(2):13–7.
29. Barros-Bailey M. The 12-step labor market survey methodology in practice: a case example. The Rehabilitation Professional 2012;20(1):1–10.
30. Van de Bittner S, Toyofuku M, Mohebbi A. Labor market survey methodology and applications. The Rehabilitation Professional 2012;20(2):119–36.
31. Baldwin M. Reducing the cost of work related musculoskeletal disorders: targeting strategies to chronic disability cases. J Electromyogr Kinesiol 2004;14(1):33–41.
32. Mayer T, Gatchel R, Polatin P, et al. Outcomes comparison of treatment for chronic disabling work-related upper-extremity disorders and spinal disorders. J Occup Environ Med 1999;41(9):761–70.
33. Power PW. A guide to vocational assessment. Austin (TX): Pro-Ed; 2006.
34. Neulicht AT, Constantini PA. The vocational expert's role in establishing damages. J Leg Nurse Consult 2002;13(3):3–10.
35. Cohen M, Yankowski T. Methodologies to improve economic and vocational analysis in personal injury litigation. Litigation Economics Digest 1996;2(1):126–35.
36. Horner SM, Slesnick F. The valuation of earning capacity definition, measurement, and evidence. J Forensic Econ 1999;12(1):13–32.
37. Alter G, Becker W. Estimating lost future earnings using the new worklife tables. Mon Labor Rev 1985;108:39–42.
38. Bureau of Labor Statistics. When one job is not enough. Available at: www.bls.gov/opub/ils/pdf/opbils40.pdf. Accessed November 10, 2012.
39. Daly P. Unpaid family workers: long-term decline continues. Mon Labor Rev 1982;105:3–5.
40. Haber S, Lamas E, Lichtenstein J. On their own: the self-employed and others in private business. Mon Labor Rev 1987;110:17–23.
41. Shaefer HL. Part-time workers: some key differences between primary and secondary earners. Mon Labor Rev 2009;132:1–15.
42. Walsh J. Myths and counter-myths: an analysis of part-time female employees and their orientations to work and working hours. Work Employ Soc 1999;13:179–203.
43. Bureau of Labor Statistics. Persons with a disability: Labor force characteristics — 2009. 2010. Available at: http://www.bls.gov/news.release/archives/disabl_08252010.pdf. Accessed November 10, 2012.
44. Foster E, Skoog G. The Markov assumption for worklife expectancy. J Forensic Econ 2004;17(2):167–83.

45. Gamboa AM, Gibson DS. The new worklife expectancy tables — revised 2006. Louisville (KY): Vocational Econometrics; 2006.

46. Ireland T. Markov process work-life expectancy tables, the LPE method for measuring worklife expectancy, and why the Gamboa-Gibson worklife expectancy tables are without merit. The Rehabilitation Professional 2009;17(3): 111–26.

47. Brookshire M, Cobb W. The life-participation-employment approach to work-life expectancy in personal injury and wrongful death cases. Defense 1983.

48. Skoog GR, Ciecka J. The Markov (increment-decrement) model of labor force activity: new results beyond worklife expectancies. J Leg Econ 2001;11(1):1–21.

49. Skoog GR, Ciecka JE, Krueger KV. The Markov process model of labor force activity: extended tables of central tendency, shape, percentile points and bootstrap standard errors. J Forensic Econ 2011;22(2):165–229.

50. Field TF, Jayne KA. Estimating worklife: BLS, Markov and disability adjustments. Estimating Earning Capacity 2008;1(2):75–99.

51. Robinson R, Spruance G. Future work propensity: a proposed alternative to purely statistical models of work-life expectancy. The Rehabilitation Professional 2011;19(1):29–36, 16.

Life Expectancy Determination

Pierre J. Vachon, PhD, JD, MPH[a],*, François Sestier, MD, PhD[b]

KEYWORDS

- Life expectancy • Mortality • Expertise • Life table • Proportional life expectancy
- Excess death rate • Relative risk

KEY POINTS

- Life expectancy is the average remaining years of survival of a group or an individual.
- Expert opinion on life expectancy must comply with evidentiary standards that apply to all expert opinion; it must be grounded in sound statistical methodology and use reliable sources of data.
- Age- and country-specific expected life expectancy data can be found in national life tables; observed excess mortality from various conditions can be found in well-selected treatises, specialized journals, medical journals, and medical textbooks.
- Excess mortality can be expressed as the difference in mortality (the excess death rates or EDRs) or by the ratio of mortality rates (MR).
- Life expectancy can be calculated by building a life table, using EDRs or MRs, or by the proportional life expectancy (PLE) method.

INTRODUCTION

Life expectancy is defined as the expected number of years left to be lived for a given person or group of people. Determining life expectancy (ie, estimating the remaining lifespan of an individual) is sometimes necessary to properly adjudicate a legal dispute. The question of life expectancy often arises when there is a need to quantify periodic payments for damages over the rest of the life of an injured or aggrieved party or when the valuation of a pension or lifelong annuity is in question (in a case of divorce, for instance). When such a case arises, the life expectancy expert will be required to perform the calculations. The expert will need to synthetize pertinent medical information and reach an opinion grounded in scientific principles and a fair application to the facts at hand. These calculations should then be presented in a clear and

Funding Sources: None to disclose.
Conflict of Interest: None to disclose.
[a] Life Expectancy Consulting, 129 Holly Terrace, Sunnyvale, CA 94086, USA; [b] Faculty of Medicine, Insurance Medicine and Medicolegal Expertise, Université de Montréal, C.P. 6128, Succursale Centre-ville, Montréal, Québec H3C 3J7, Canada
* Corresponding author.
E-mail address: vachon@lifeexpectancyexpert.net

Phys Med Rehabil Clin N Am 24 (2013) 539–551
http://dx.doi.org/10.1016/j.pmr.2013.03.007
1047-9651/13/$ – see front matter © 2013 Elsevier Inc. All rights reserved.

relevant format so they can be used by other experts such as life care planners, economists, and actuaries.[1] This article discusses some of the important aspects of determining life expectancy and the principles employed to formulate expert opinion on life expectancy.

DEFINITION

Life expectancy is a mathematical concept applied to survival; it is defined as the average remaining years of survival for a group or an individual. It is sometimes confused with, but is distinct from, the median survival time (ie, the expected age at which half of the individuals in a population will have died). Life expectancy may generally approach the same value as median survival time, but it remains a fundamentally different concept. It should also be underscored that life expectancy refers to the remaining years to be lived, not the expected age at death. Confusion abounds on this, because the only widely disseminated information on life expectancy is what is properly called, but almost never is, "life expectancy at birth." Thus, the life expectancy of a 50-year-old man will never be 80, for example, but it could very well be, say, 30 years.

Given that life expectancy is by definition a projection, inherent in its calculation is some hypothesis about the future of mortality. Most often, the hypothesis is that the current state of mortality—the mortality observable at the time of the projection— will remain constant forever. The soundness of this hypothesis is of course debatable, but in the context of calculations for litigation, it is by far the most popular assumption, as it does not involve complicated projection models about the evolution of mortality patterns. (Some jurisdictions may dictate the hypotheses to be employed. For instance, British courts will mandate that a schedule of projected (evolving) mortality rates be used[2]). Using a collection of age-specific mortality rates, it is possible to apply straightforward calculations to generate a complete life table comprising the future probabilities of survival at each age, the person-years lived in each age range, and the life expectancy at each age, among other quantities.[3,4]

BASIC NOTIONS

Some have claimed that estimating life expectancy for an individual is impossible, as the very concept applies only to a group. This is not a sound argument, given that the principle of statistical inference is valid. Moreover, often this spurious claim is immediately followed by the proposal that the general population life table be used instead of the expert's calculation, thus defeating the very argument. The theoretical notion of group is, however, important to the concept of life expectancy. To reach a reasonable opinion, the expert needs to identify and discern a group of people that fits the profile of the individual. In theory, the expert would want the match to be perfect on all significant parameters. This usually starts with age, sex, nationality, and sometimes race; the expert would then add the specific medical information pertinent to the individual. In practice, the data available in the real world are limited. The expert will therefore try to match the available data to the individual in question as best as practically and reasonably possible to ensure that the mortality rates employed in calculations truly reflect the expected mortality profile of the individual (For example, an individual with coronary artery disease might be matched on the number of affected vessels, the ejection fraction, and perhaps even the concentration of N-terminal probrain natriuretic peptide (NT-proBNP), a biomarker used to estimate cardiovascular disease risk). Once a group is identified, it is possible to calculate, estimate, and extrapolate life expectancy based on the data pertaining to the known group.

Survival of individuals in the group will of course vary; some people will live longer, and some will live shorter. But in the absence of information, variables, or parameters that allow the expert to make a statistically grounded distinction among the individuals in the group, imputing the group average to all individuals is the best policy. The average is in such cases an unbiased estimator.

ABOUT EXPERTISE

An opinion on life expectancy prepared for the court will need to comport with well-established evidentiary standards. In the United States, these are the rules either of Daubert or Frye, depending on the jurisdiction (federal courts and most states have adopted the standards put forth by the Supreme Court of the United States in *Daubert v Merrell Dow Pharmaceuticals*. Some states retain the standards of *Frye v United States*). Among the factors the court will consider when assessing admissibility are whether the method has been subject to peer review and publication, the existence of standards and controls for the method, and the degree to which the method has been accepted by the relevant scientific community. The method outlined in this article meets those requirements and has been accepted by numerous courts in the United States, Canada, United Kingdom, and Australia. In contrast, several purported methods fail on all prongs of the Daubert test. Among the methods to be avoided is the deduction of a fixed number of years for any given medical condition (Because the mathematics of life tables is nonlinear, this direct but simplistic attempt necessarily fails, despite the claims of some[5]). Defaulting to the general population life expectancy (usually on the grounds that the general population contains everyone and is therefore an appropriate estimate for anyone) also should be avoided (The general population life expectancy is appropriate when differentiating factors are not known. However, if some factors are known and present in the individual, the general population is no longer an appropriate estimate. As an illustration, the mean annual income in the United States is a general average. If one wants to estimate the expected annual income of a Fortune 500 chief executive officer (CEO), the general US mean is inappropriate even if all CEOs are included in the larger average. The fact that they are CEOs makes them a distinct subgroup with its own average). Additionally, declaratory statements based on nothing more than nonsystematic data, such as from personal clinical experience should be avoided. Similarly, statements to the effect that an individual could live to a normal life expectancy or that the average of a subgroup does not apply to the individual because of alleged but not demonstrably distinguishing characteristics should not be credited, as they merely betray a misunderstanding of the very concept of life expectancy.

Experts in general must be qualified by education, training, or experience. In the case of life expectancy, the expert must be knowledgeable about and adept at statistics. Typically, although perhaps not exclusively, this will mean graduate-level education in statistics, biostatistics, epidemiology, demography, or actuarial science. Although statistical knowledge is the only requirement per se, an individual wishing to qualify as an expert for life expectancy would be well advised to possess some knowledge of medicine, or, failing that, retain the services of qualified assistants.

SOURCES OF DATA

The most often-used data are the national life tables. These tables would be appropriate if the only information known about a patient was age, sex, and nationality. Here, the match of the individual to the group would be perfect (same age, sex, and nationality). If any medical condition is involved, however, the expert needs to take into account any excess mortality that may apply. Data on the excess mortality of various conditions can be found in treatises, specialized journals, medical journals, and medical textbooks. But even then, it will probably be necessary to make some use of base mortality rates, usually from national tables. These are most often produced by national statistical agencies and are easily obtainable. In the United States, the tables published by the Centers for Disease Control and Prevention (CDC)[6] are certainly adequate. Sometimes, other organizations may hold collections of life tables derived from official data[7]; a cursory look at their methodological specifications should suffice to ascertain the value of such tables. Some even estimate data at the subnational level.[8] However, employing these tables rather than national tables would probably be advisable only after verifying the jurisdictional requirements.

MATHEMATICS OF LIFE EXPECTANCY

Life expectancy cannot, for practical reasons, be measured directly. This would entail waiting for everyone in the whole group of interest to die (Note that, when preoccupied with historical matters, such tables are compiled upon extinction. These life tables are called cohort life tables, in contrast with the much more common period life tables). The way to measure life expectancy is to calculate age-specific mortality rates. It should be noted that although rates and probabilities are related concepts, they are not the same quantity, and although it is possible to calculate life expectancy based on age-specific probabilities of death, mortality rates are preferable for technical reasons that will be explained. Life expectancy is calculated by amalgamating a series of age-specific mortality rates to replicate the mortality experience of a whole life span. Applying this series of rates to a theoretical population yields a set of survival probabilities at each age. For example, one can calculate the 1-year mortality rate of people age 20 by relating the number of deaths occurring in a given year to people between 20 and 21 to the number of 20-year-olds alive during that year (for national tables, this is done using census data and death records). For a given year, this is done for all ages. Thus, as an example, the life table for Canadian females in 2007 (**Table 1**) will be constructed using a collection of age-specific mortality rates from ages 0 to over 100, each of which was calculated on the basis of the number of observed deaths between ages x and x + 1 and the estimated population of people aged x, for x in values of 0 to the maximum age of the life table.

Table 1 shows an abridged (abridged here refers to both the omission of data actually employed in the calculation and the truncation at age 100. The former means that values were calculated for each annual age, despite only decennial ages being shown for ages greater than 20. These data are omitted from the output only to make the final table easier to view. The latter, however, involves real data censoring. The genuine data for ages 100 and beyond were collapsed into a singular category of 100+). The term lx is the number of survivors at the corresponding age, and dx is the number of people dying at that age in the life table. The terms qx and mx stand for the probability of death and the mortality rate at age x, respectively. The probability of death is merely dx/lx. The term mx, the mortality rate, is defined as the number of deaths over person-years lived. This latter quantity is labeled Lx; it is the number of years lived in the interval from x to x + 1. It is equal to the sum of people alive at the beginning of the interval who survive all the way to the end (ie, those who were alive and survived over the interval) multiplied by 1 (the duration of the interval), and the product of those dying in the interval (dx) by their average length of survival in the interval (labeled ax, and a variable almost always equal to 0.5) (At age 0, deaths are severely skewed toward the first days of life. Accordingly, deaths at age 0 do not in fact occur at an average age of

Table 1
Abridged life table, Canada, females, 2007

Age	lx	dx	mx	qx	ax	Lx	Tx	ex
0	100,000	477	0.00478	0.00477	0.07	99,557	8,295,368	82.95
1	99,523	29	0.00029	0.00029	0.5	99,509	8,195,811	82.35
2	99,494	19	0.00019	0.00019	0.5	99,485	8,096,303	81.37
3	99,475	10	0.00010	0.00010	0.5	99,470	7,996,818	80.39
4	99,465	10	0.00010	0.00010	0.5	99,460	7,897,347	79.40
5	99,455	14	0.00014	0.00014	0.5	99,449	7,797,887	78.41
6	99,442	13	0.00013	0.00013	0.5	99,435	7,698,438	77.42
7	99,429	14	0.00014	0.00014	0.5	99,422	7,599,003	76.43
8	99,415	10	0.00010	0.00010	0.5	99,410	7,499,582	75.44
9	99,405	10	0.00010	0.00010	0.5	99,400	7,400,172	74.44
10	99,395	7	0.00007	0.00007	0.5	99,391	7,300,772	73.45
11	99,388	8	0.00008	0.00008	0.5	99,384	7,201,381	72.46
12	99,380	11	0.00011	0.00011	0.5	99,374	7,101,997	71.46
13	99,369	11	0.00011	0.00011	0.5	99,364	7,002,622	70.47
14	99,358	18	0.00018	0.00018	0.5	99,349	6,903,259	69.48
15	99,340	21	0.00021	0.00021	0.5	99,330	6,803,910	68.49
16	99,319	20	0.00020	0.00020	0.5	99,309	6,704,580	67.51
17	99,299	26	0.00026	0.00026	0.5	99,287	6,605,270	66.52
18	99,274	34	0.00034	0.00034	0.5	99,257	6,505,984	65.54
19	99,240	31	0.00031	0.00031	0.5	99,225	6,406,727	64.56
20	99,209	30	0.00030	0.00030	0.5	99,194	6,307,503	63.58
30	98,902	36	0.00036	0.00036	0.5	98,884	5,316,914	53.76
40	98,401	78	0.00079	0.00079	0.5	98,362	4,330,091	44.00
50	97,050	217	0.00224	0.00224	0.5	96,942	3,351,702	34.54
60	93,842	514	0.00549	0.00547	0.5	93,585	2,395,083	25.52
70	86,337	1190	0.01388	0.01378	0.5	85,742	1,488,783	17.24
80	69,102	2583	0.03810	0.03738	0.5	67,811	700,495	10.14
90	33,896	4045	0.12707	0.11933	0.5	31,873	170,019	5.02
100+	3615	3615	0.41254	1.00000	0.5	8763	8763	2.42

Data from The human mortality database. University of California, Berkeley (USA), and Max Planck Institute for Demographic Research (Germany). Available at: www.mortality.org or www.humanmortality.de. Accessed October 1, 2012.

0.5 years. At the very last age, the collapsing of several ages into a singular category also affects a_x). So $m_x = d_x/L_x$. The value T_x is the same as all remaining L_x, from age x to the end of life. The term e_x is the life expectancy, calculated as T_x/l_x.

From a purely mathematical standpoint, the calculations used to build a life table resemble those used when calculating compound interest, only in reverse. The calculation starts with a beginning amount (initial population) and applies successive interest rates (mortality rates), which increase (decrease) the amount (population) with every time period. Consequently, the numbers involved do not vary linearly; life expectancy cannot be calculated by simply adjusting the total upwards or downwards by fixed values for given conditions. It also means that linear interpolation is technically incorrect. Although linear interpolation may be of little or no consequence over small intervals (eg, between 27.2 and 27.8 years), the midpoint of life expectancies between

20 and 30 is not a life expectancy of 25. Similarly, halving of mortality rates does not double life expectancy. Simply put, there is no shortcut, and life expectancy must be calculated with a full set of mortality rates built into a life table.

DIAGNOSIS AND MEDICAL EVALUATION

If no medical information is available on the individual, the expert would simply employ the general population life table. For a nonstandard individual, however, it will be necessary to ascertain the condition or conditions that may cause the need for a distinct analysis. An assessment of the medical situation of the individual is usually achieved through 1 of 2 ways: a comprehensive and thorough review of the individual's medical records, or an independent medical examination. If both are feasible, it may be best to combine the approaches, as medical records may not completely reflect the current status of the individual, and an examination may not reveal past medical events of significance.

The purpose of the diagnosis is to identify the conditions that are relevant to calculating life expectancy. This raises the question which conditions matter. This determination arises by reviewing the literature; in turn, as will be described, the literature review is guided by the diagnosis. Experience with actual calculations of life expectancy and previous considerations of technical articles on the several medical diagnoses of the patient render the expert capable of assessing which conditions will be important for the ultimate opinion.

To ascertain which medical conditions are present, the expert will most often rely on evaluations performed by others; the most useful is probably the independent medical examination, especially if conducted for the dispute at hand. A thorough review of medical records is also indicated to acquire a long-term view of the patient's medical profile, but also to gather information about all potential items affecting life expectancy. Finally, in cases where the expert is asked for the hypothetical life expectancy of a deceased individual (often in a lawsuit for torts, where the plaintiff alleges that negligence caused the death, and that compensation is owed in some fashion related to the lifespan of the deceased), the autopsy report can contain precious information evaluated by an independent source.

AN ESSENTIAL STEP: THE LITERATURE REVIEW

How does the expert know whether a given medical condition is associated with increased mortality? Expert opinion must be grounded in sound scientific principles, and the expert opinion on life expectancy is no exception. Subjective perception based on general experience is most likely insufficient to support a conclusion in this context. The vast expanse of medical literature contains a tremendous amount of information, and in all likelihood a detailed study has been published on the medical condition in question.

A summary search of the literature (eg, PubMed contains more than 22 million citations from the biomedical literature[9]) will in most cases reveal that several articles have been published from which the expert can derive suitable mortality rates. For almost any condition, the aggregation of the results from several studies will generate data that are much more valuable to correctly ascertain mortality than the clinical judgment and experience of even a specialized practitioner. The rigors of peer review make it so that published data are strictly and systematically collected and analyzed; casual clinical data, however seemingly plentiful, are no substitute if they were not gathered in a fashion that would pass muster with academic reviewers. One should also resist the lure of relying on a singular, groundbreaking study in the face of an otherwise broad consensus in the literature. Revolutions in treatment and survival can and do occur, but the possibility of an outlier study should be considered. Random statistical deviations in studies with small sample sizes, poor study methodology, and low generalizability are all possibilities the expert should keep in mind.

When assessing the relative value of several studies on a given topic, be mindful of certain factors that tend to correlate with higher quality and reliability. First and foremost, the size and type of study are of tremendous importance. Case–control studies will usually be small and of little use. Randomized control trials may he gold standard of medical research, but their often tight inclusion criteria may limit the generalizability of the results to the general population. Optimally, a large cohort study with very long follow-up would prove better. A well-designed meta-analysis can also provide valuable information, because, in effect, a proper review of literature will seek to integrate into the expert opinion as many pertinent studies as possible; a well-conducted meta-analysis is just a shortcut to what ultimately needs to be done. Reaching a conclusion as to the mortality associated with a condition will require that the expert exert some judgment in the face of multiple studies, not all of which will yield the same results. Ultimately, the opinion should discuss the findings from the literature review and acknowledge and justify any selection or judgment calls.

Some specialized sources may also contain the mortality rates associated with certain conditions for the specific purpose of calculating survival. Such sources are usually the product of solid research on condition-specific mortality, and can save much research time. They include manuals,[10] certain Web sites pertaining to legal medicine and insurance matters,[11] and the rating manuals of life insurance and reinsurance companies.

GOOD DATA

It would be ideal if medical journals were rife with articles directly addressing life expectancy. For some conditions, reliable studies have been published that greatly facilitate the task of the expert. In fact, if one finds such an article, it may be of sufficient quality and detail to enable a nonexpert to directly estimate life expectancy. But even then, the data that life care planners and economists require for their purposes are usually a full life table, and those are almost inexistent in the literature. The data the expert needs to find are mortality rates, or other data that allow for the calculation of mortality rates. Most often, this will be in the form of survival probabilities, relative risks, or survival curves. Ideally, a peer-reviewed article with a large sample population would be preferable, since larger samples yield more stable and reliable measurements. The data should be transparent as to the selection process (ie, which individuals were excluded or included in the study population). The expert needs clear information on the age, sex, medical condition, comorbidities, and, of course, survival. The expert would also want, if applicable, stratified data for levels, grades, or intensities of the medical condition. A narrower subgroup allows for a more precise matching to the individual and consequently to a more accurate estimate of life expectancy. For example, individuals with type 2 diabetes mellitus with neuropathy comprise a more precise group than the much broader group of all diabetic patients, or individuals with coronary artery disease of 3 vessels with reduced ejection fraction comprise a narrower group than those with heart disease.

TRADEOFFS AND PRAGMATISM

Practical considerations will sometimes force a choice between robustness and precision. A larger study with more cases could produce results that are more suitable than a study with a narrowly defined subset of the condition but statistically uncertain estimates of the mortality rates. Or, sometimes, a very good study will be available for a different age group, the opposite sex, or a population in a different country. This can be frustrating, even though some methods can correct for such factors. And, sometimes, multiple studies contemplating the same condition for comparable patients will yield mutually incoherent results. The expert must then try to square the results as researchers do when conducting meta-analyses. Statistical methods can be of succor for this, but the technical judgment of an experienced epidemiologist may prove useful in assessing the relative value of such studies.

CALCULATION ILLUSTRATED

To show the process of life expectancy calculation, consider the following hypothetical case. An expert is asked to calculate the life expectancy of a 50-year-old Canadian woman with presumed moderate-to-severe medical conditions. A review of the medical records reveals a history of conditions X, Y, and Z, but the current state of Z is uncertain, since the records are somewhat dated. An independent medical examination is performed that reveals X is ongoing but stable; Y is worse than the records indicated, and Z seems to have resolved. The examination also identifies previously undetected condition W. With this in mind, the expert should search the literature to determine whether these conditions have a bearing on survival. The search reveals that a current condition of Z may be detrimental but that a history of Z is not. Also, the literature on W suggests that no excess mortality is associated with the condition. The expert's experience with other cases and condition X has shown that several reliable articles detail the mortality experience of men about that age with condition X. The excess mortality is constant and equal to 0.005.

The search, however, identifies only 2 articles addressing condition Y. One is a large double-blind multicenter intervention study of about 3000 patients with condition Y with an average age of 40 years, while the other is a small observational study of 100 cases of Y in women aged about 50 years in a single medical facility. In such a situation, if the studies do not entirely agree, it would probably be preferable to base the opinion on the first study, given its nature (a double-blind study could very well have tighter controls) and given the much larger number of patients. Sample size matters for 2 reasons; it makes it more likely that disease severity is stratified on a gradient, and that the resulting estimates are statistically more stable with smaller standard errors. Note that it would certainly be reasonable to conduct a regression analysis on the data to give some weight to both studies, although weighing the results would be warranted.

Once such raw data have been garnered, the expert would extract from these articles the mortality rates or survival probabilities. The reported data usually require some mathematical manipulation. For instance, if 1-year survival is 97%, the probability of death would simply be 3%, but the mortality rate would be $(-1) \times \ln(0.97) = 0.03046$. Similarly, if a given 5-year survival is 88%, the annual mortality rate is $[(-1) \times \ln(0.88)]/5 = 0.1278/5 = 0.02557$. Once this rate is obtained for a specific age and sex, the expert looks to the expected mortality at that age; this is the mortality that would be expected in a person similar in all ways save for the presence of the medical condition. Such data are obtained from national, provincial, or state tables for the general population. In this case, the expert would seek the life table for Canadian females, and note the mortality rate labeled mx for age 50. This value, as per the life table (**Table 2**) is 0.00224. Using the value derived from the 5-year survival, the mortality differential is calculated in 1 of 2 ways: either as an absolute difference or

Table 2
Abridged table of mortality rates for 50-year-old Canadian women with conditions X and Y: base rate, rate for condition X, rate for condition Y, and total rate

Age	Base Rate	Rate for X	Rate for Y	Total Rate
50	0.00224	0.005	0.02333	0.03057
51	0.00233	0.005	0.02397	0.03130
52	0.00275	0.005	0.02465	0.03240
53	0.00288	0.005	0.02535	0.03324
54	0.00305	0.005	0.02610	0.03415
55	0.00330	0.005	0.02689	0.03519
56	0.00375	0.005	0.02772	0.03647
57	0.00411	0.005	0.02860	0.03771
58	0.00452	0.005	0.02953	0.03905
59	0.00469	0.005	0.03051	0.04020
60	0.00549	0.005	0.03156	0.04205
61	0.00545	0.005	0.03266	0.04311
62	0.00600	0.005	0.03386	0.04486
63	0.00695	0.005	0.03512	0.04707
64	0.00795	0.005	0.03646	0.04942
65	0.00834	0.005	0.03788	0.05123
66	0.00912	0.005	0.03941	0.05353
67	0.01035	0.005	0.04105	0.05640
68	0.01164	0.005	0.04280	0.05944
69	0.01207	0.005	0.04466	0.06173
70	0.01388	0.005	0.04669	0.06557
71	0.01537	0.005	0.04886	0.06923
72	0.01664	0.005	0.05119	0.07283
73	0.01779	0.005	0.05373	0.07653
74	0.02030	0.005	0.05652	0.08182
75	0.02191	0.005	0.05952	0.08643
76	0.02440	0.005	0.06281	0.09221
77	0.02768	0.005	0.06641	0.09909
78	0.03002	0.005	0.07031	0.10534
79	0.03468	0.005	0.07465	0.11432
80	0.03810	0.005	0.07932	0.12242
90	0.12708	0.005	0.15905	0.29113
100	0.35939	0.005	0.28972	0.65410

as a ratio. So, combining these examples, if one had a Canadian woman aged 50 years with a particular condition, and reliable references in the medical literature documenting a 5-year survival of 88% for Canadian women aged about 50 years with the condition, one can perform some calculations to estimate the mortality rate over the life course. The absolute differential is called the excess death rate or EDR[12]; it would here be equal for age 50 to 0.02557–0.00224 = 0.02333. The ratio is usually called the relative risk or RR, but is sometimes also called the risk ratio. It would here be equal to 0.02557/0.00224 = 11.415. The expert would calculate these values for each of the conditions in a case with multiple ailments.

With these tools, the mortality rate can now be calculated for an individual of age 50 years with all of the previously mentioned conditions at once. This is performed by either adding all the EDRs (1 for each condition) to the base mortality rate of the general population, or by multiplying the base rate by the sum of RRs. Summing EDRs is straightforward. The total EDR is just the sum of the component EDRs: $EDR_1 + EDR_2 + \ldots = $ (total EDR). Consolidating several RRs into 1 RR value is slightly trickier: one needs to subtract 1 from each individual RR value, after which they can be summed: $(RR_1 - 1) + (RR_2 - 1) + \ldots + 1 = $ (total RR). The mx value for 50 with the condition is equal to mx (50) + (total EDR) or mx (50) × (total RR). Both yield the same value at that age.

Such a calculation produces a result for only 1 year of the individual's age, and one needs a complete series of mortality rates for all ages up to the terminal age (usually 100). With this singular age-specific mortality rate, methods are available to estimate all the other age-specific rates for the given profile of the patient. Two methods stand out as more precise and accurate than others: 1 based on EDRs and 1 based on RRs. Both will lead to a valid opinion, although they diverge slightly in their ultimate outcomes.[13] The method of proportional life expectancy (PLE) was employed to calculate the series of mortality rates for condition Y in **Table 2**.

Armed with a complete series of mortality rates, the expert can now build a life table. The method is very much standard. A theoretical arbitrary population, usually 100,000 or 10,000, is put through the gauntlet of successive mortality rates. If 100,000 Canadian women aged 50 years with medical conditions X and Y were followed for a year, one would expect $(100,000) \times e^{-0.3011} = 96,989$ to be alive at age 51. Thus, 3011 would die in the first year. The total person-years lived in that first interval would be equal to $(96,989 + 3011/2) = 98,495$, the value of Lx. This is repeated for all ages, up to 100. From this series of survivors at each age, one can compute the life expectancy. But it is in fact those numbers of survivors that will be employed in calculations by the life care planner or the economist. This is why it is essential to build a complete life table and not merely report the life expectancy. It is entirely possible that 2 different patients with the same life expectancy could have different profiles of expected survival at each age, with a mere coincident that the averages happen to be equal. Just like a 50–50 chance of winning 10 or 0, and a 50–50 chance of winning 4 or 6 both have an expected value of 5, life expectancies alone can hide considerable variability in the underlying distribution of survival. A full table ensures proper valuation, if such is needed; the nonlinear aspects of life expectancy, just as with compound interest rates, mandate that each age-specific survival proportion be considered, not just the average. The resulting life table corresponding to the authors' example is shown in **Table 3**. One can see from **Table 3** that the life expectancy at age 50 is about 18.1. If a person with this profile were to reach age 60, the life expectancy at that point would then be about 13.6.

LIMITATIONS

For all its mathematical precision, the validity of a life expectancy calculation nonetheless rests on several assumptions that may prove inaccurate. Foremost, it presumes a stable state of mortality. That is, the mortality that prevails today is presumed to remain the same in the future, sometimes for several decades. On its face, this proposition seems somewhat ludicrous, as medical knowledge and technology progress with time. But 3 reasons exist to forego correcting or adjusting for future advances and expected decreases in mortality. First, it is not certain that such advances will materialize. This may seem pessimistic, but the steady advances in survival could

Table 3
Abridged life table for 50-year-old Canadian women with conditions X and Y

Age	lx	dx	mx	qx	Lx	Tx	ex
50	100,000	3011	0.03011	0.03057	98,495	1,810,023	18.10
51	96,989	2989	0.03082	0.03130	95,495	1,711,529	17.65
52	94,001	2997	0.03188	0.03240	92,502	1,616,034	17.19
53	91,004	2975	0.03269	0.03324	89,517	1,523,531	16.74
54	88,029	2956	0.03357	0.03415	86,551	1,434,015	16.29
55	85,074	2942	0.03458	0.03519	83,603	1,347,463	15.84
56	82,132	2942	0.03582	0.03647	80,661	1,263,861	15.39
57	79,190	2931	0.03701	0.03771	77,725	1,183,200	14.94
58	76,259	2920	0.03829	0.03905	74,799	1,105,475	14.50
59	73,339	2890	0.03941	0.04020	71,894	1,030,676	14.05
60	70,449	2901	0.04118	0.04205	68,998	958,782	13.61
61	67,548	2850	0.04220	0.04311	66,123	889,783	13.17
62	64,698	2838	0.04387	0.04486	63,279	823,660	12.73
63	61,860	2844	0.04598	0.04707	60,437	760,382	12.29
64	59,015	2845	0.04822	0.04942	57,592	699,944	11.86
65	56,170	2805	0.04994	0.05123	54,767	642,352	11.44
66	53,365	2781	0.05212	0.05353	51,974	587,584	11.01
67	50,584	2774	0.05484	0.05640	49,196	535,610	10.59
68	47,809	2759	0.05771	0.05944	46,430	486,414	10.17
69	45,051	2697	0.05986	0.06173	43,702	439,984	9.77
70	42,354	2688	0.06347	0.06557	41,010	396,282	9.36
71	39,666	2653	0.06688	0.06923	38,339	355,272	8.96
72	37,013	2600	0.07024	0.07283	35,713	316,933	8.56
73	34,413	2535	0.07367	0.07653	33,145	281,220	8.17
74	31,878	2504	0.07856	0.08182	30,625	248,075	7.78
75	29,373	2432	0.08280	0.08643	28,157	217,449	7.40
76	26,941	2373	0.08809	0.09221	25,755	189,292	7.03
77	24,568	2318	0.09434	0.09909	23,409	163,537	6.66
78	22,250	2225	0.09998	0.10534	21,138	140,128	6.30
79	20,026	2163	0.10803	0.11432	18,944	118,990	5.94
80	17,862	2058	0.11522	0.12242	16,833	100,046	5.60
90	2785	704	0.25258	0.29113	2434	7918	2.84
100+	32	32	0.51135	1.00000	24	62	1.96

be seriously hampered by either catastrophic events or prolonged behavioral or environmental changes that temporarily or permanently change the mortality landscape. The rise in the prevalence of obesity, for example, could very well prove to be detrimental to future life spans. The second reason has to do with uncertainty. Even if a decline in future mortality rates was certain, the precise pace or extent of decline may remain uncertain. What values would then be used, given that opinions offered as expertise cannot be based on pure speculation?

The third reason is much more pragmatic, and some would argue much more compelling. The rules of evidence dictate to some extent the parameters. An expert cannot in all cases simply introduce conjecture about the future state of the world.

Much like an economist may be constrained to use the current prevailing interest rate, the life expectancy expert may be limited to employing current, measurable, observable, and somewhat tangible mortality rates. The rules need not be this way, of course, and some jurisdictions, such as in the UK, mandate the use of projected rates—ie, rates that vary over time in the future. But it is beyond the scope of the expertise to try to change the rules of the court and compliance is indicated.

Another limitation is in the assumption of independence. When a patient suffers from multiple conditions, to what extent are any of them duplicative? That is, if someone suffers from obesity, hypertension, coronary artery disease, and diabetes mellitus, it would be unwise to simply cumulate all the risks measured individually. To some extent, the excess mortality from diabetes mellitus or hypertension is related to heart disease. To count each risk individually and then sum all of them would certainly factor in significant double or triple counting. An individual should not be taxed several times for what are in fact several risks overlapping and somewhat blending into one.

The expert could, of course, try to identify a study or article addressing survival for patients with this particular complex of pathologies, but this may prove fruitless. In such cases, some epidemiologic judgment may be called for as to which risks are independent and which overlap partially or completely. In some rare cases, the global risk may actually be greater than the sum of the parts, when some synergy between the risks exists (for instance, it may be so that the excess mortality associated with smoking and asbestos exposure is greater than the sum of each individual risk). In complex cases like these, the exercise of calculation is not simply formulaic. If independent judgment may, or should, be exercised in such complicated cases, it is of course no license to jettison any relation to scientific foundations. Complexity does not grant a license to speculate groundlessly; the opinion must remain within the realm of the epidemiologically sound.

THE REPORT

Because the purpose of life expectancy opinion is to inform the courts and other experts, it should be presented in a clear and straightforward way that makes its use by other experts as easy as possible. This entails presenting not only the scalar value of life expectancy but also the expected distribution of survival times (ie, the life table). However, given that the opinion must comport with standards of evidence and of science, the foundations of the opinions should also be laid out, probably as a preamble to the opinion, so that all parties involved and fellow experts can assess, evaluate, critique, and even reproduce the calculations.

A life expectancy report should therefore state the facts on which the opinion is based, and when necessary, the sources used (eg, medical records or findings from an independent medical examination). It should also identify the textbooks, rating manual, or academic journal articles on which the expert relied. It should provide an explanation of the hypotheses or assumptions underlying the calculations and adjustments. It should then describe the calculations performed with sufficient detail as to enable reproduction of the results by a sufficiently qualified expert in the field. Last, it should present the results in the form of a life table (or several life tables, if hypothetical scenarios are considered) so as to enable any valuation dependent on year-by-year survival probabilities.

SUMMARY

An expert opinion on life expectancy should comply with the standards that apply to expertise in general. The opinion needs to be rooted in reasonable factual assumptions and appropriate and reliable technical methods. The expert should first inquire if a valid diagnosis was made, and if all the information that may be required is sustained by valid evidence. The expert must not cherry-pick facts or diagnoses. Care must be taken that a proper comparison group is constituted, and reasonable judgment should be exercised in the selection of the studies employed to calculate mortality rates; the assessment of the technical literature must be neutral and fair. A clear and detailed report should be produced, containing the basis for the opinion, the description of the methods employed, and the specific calculations performed. And, last, the report should be designed in such a way that it informs and enlightens, but does not advocate. The function of expert opinion is not to persuade, but rather to help the decision maker.

REFERENCES

1. Singer RB. How to prepare a life expectancy report for an attorney in a tort case. J Insur Med 2005;37:42–51.
2. Government Actuary's Department. Actuarial tables with explanatory notes for use in personal injury and fatal accident cases. 7th edition. Available at: www.gad.gov.uk/Documents/Other%20Services/Ogden%20Tables/Ogden_Tables_7th_edition.pdf. Accessed October 1, 2012.
3. Keyfitz N, Caswell H. Applied mathematical demography. 3rd edition. New York: Springer Science, Business Media; 2005.
4. London D. Survival models and their estimation. 3rd edition. Winsted (CT): Actex Publications; 1997.
5. Thomas R, Barnes M. Life expectancy for people with disabilities. NeuroRehabilitation 2010;27:201–9.
6. Arias E. United States Life Tables, 2007. National Vital Statistics Reports. US Dept. of Health and Human Services; 2011. p. 1–61. Available at: www.cdc.gov/nchs/data/nvsr/nvsr59/nvsr59_09.pdf. Accessed October 1, 2012.
7. The human mortality database. Available at: www.mortality.org. Accessed October 1, 2012.
8. Canadian human mortality database. Available at: www.bdlc.umontreal.ca/CHMD. Accessed October 1, 2012.
9. National Center for Biotechnology Information, U.S. National Library of Medicine. PubMed. Available at: www.ncbi.nlm.nih.gov/pubmed. Accessed October 1, 2012.
10. Brackenridge RD, Croxson RS, MacKenzie BR, editors. Brackenridge's medical selection of life risks. 5th edition. New York: Palgrave Macmillan; 2006.
11. Université de Montréal. Program in insurance medicine and medicolegal expertise. Available at: www.mae.umontreal.ca/. Accessed October 1, 2012.
12. Singer RB. A method of relating life expectancy in the US population life table to excess mortality. J Insur Med 1992;24:32–41.
13. Strauss DJ, Vachon PJ, Shavelle RM. Estimation of future mortality rates and life expectancy in chronic medical conditions. J Insur Med 2005;37:20–34.

Published Research and Physiatric Opinion in Life Care Planning

Reg L. Gibbs, MS, CRC, LCPC, CBIS, CLCP[a,b,*], Bill S. Rosen, MD[c],
Michel Lacerte, MDCM, MSc, FRCPC, CCRC[d,e]

KEYWORDS

- Evidence-based recommendations • Life care planning • Literature search
- Literature review • Medicolegal ethics • Code of conduct

KEY POINTS

- Providing life care planners with evidence-based recommendations requires a thorough knowledge of how to search, read, and critically apply literature findings to the individual patient.
- Knowledge of available databases, as well as how to determine the relevancy and validity of research findings, is key to providing evidence-based recommendations.
- The physiatrist performing medicolegal work must be aware of their ethical duties.

INTRODUCTION

The soundness of any life care plan depends on how thoroughly it addresses an individual patient's or client's needs. Accuracy in a life care plan requires establishing a proper foundation of opinion for recommended services. Physiatrists who provide expert opinion for life care plans should be guided by the recognition that recommendations for the long-term needs of permanently injured or impaired persons must be based solidly on medical evidence. In turn, the life care planner should incorporate the physiatrist's recommendations in a comprehensive manner and be consistent in

Funding Sources: None.
Conflict of Interest: R.L. Gibbs: owner of Brightsun Technologies, the company that created FormPro. B.S. Rosen, M. Lacerte: none.
[a] Rocky Mountain Rehab, Brightsun Technologies Inc, PO Box 20253, Billings, MT 59104, USA;
[b] Montana State University-Billings, Billings, MT, USA; [c] Montana Neuroscience Institute, Montana Brain Injury Center, St. Patrick Hospital, 1637 South Higgins Avenue, Missoula, MT 59801, USA; [d] Department of Physical Medicine & Rehabilitation, Schulich School of Medicine and Dentistry, Western University, Box 10, Lambeth Station, London, Ontario N6P 1P9, Canada; [e] Insurance Medicine and Medico-legal Expertise Diploma Program, Université de Montréal Faculté de Médecine, C.P. 6128, Succursale Centre-ville, Montréal, Québec H3C 3J7, Canada
* Corresponding author. Brightsun Technologies Inc, PO Box 20253, Billings, MT 59104.
E-mail address: rgibbs@brightsuntech.com

Phys Med Rehabil Clin N Am 24 (2013) 553–566
http://dx.doi.org/10.1016/j.pmr.2013.03.002
1047-9651/13/$ – see front matter © 2013 Elsevier Inc. All rights reserved.

his or her methodology. The physiatrist providing recommendations to the life care planner can help bolster his or her opinion on the long-term care needs of the individual by applying findings from relevant, peer-reviewed literature. Fundamental elements of evidence-based life care planning include a commitment to a frequent review of relevant literature to stay informed about current research, as well as developing criteria for determining research acceptability.[1] Advantages of evidence-based life care planning include defensibility of opinions given in plans and in testimony, the minimization of errors and omissions in determining care needs, and better treatment guidelines for patients to follow, leading to optimal medical and rehabilitation outcomes.

SEARCHING THE LITERATURE

A variety of databases index literature useful in determining long-term care needs and research related to life care planning. Examples of such databases include the following:

- CINAHL via EBSCOhost: a database of more than 3000 journals for nursing and allied health research, with more than 610 being free full-text titles[2]
- APA PsycNET: a database that indexes and delivers American Psychological Association content and offers institutional site licenses as well as individual access to articles on behavioral science research[3]
- PubMed: a free database that primarily accesses MEDLINE, a database of references and abstracts on the life sciences and biomedical topics; PubMed contains more than 22 million records for biomedical literature[4]
- Elsevier: a publishing company that publishes around 1250 journals and close to 20,000 books and major reference texts related to science and health information[5]

Another database resource for physiatrists and life care planners is FormPro,[6] a resource created by Reg Gibbs, one of the authors of this article. This database is designed specifically to collect evidence-based information on a variety of common diagnoses that are often encountered when preparing a life care plan. The articles cited in FormPro focus on the long-term care needs of the individual. FormPro includes peer-reviewed articles and resources that pertain to such needs and can be searched by keyword, injury type, and pediatric and adult age groups. FormPro's database includes journal articles, books, clinical practice guidelines, and Web sites that provide evidence to support case-related recommendations. FormPro is a valuable resource for life care planners and medical professionals commenting on long-term care needs, because the database screens out research that is not relevant or of good quality, such as studies on animals and studies on acute care needs or treatment strategies for individuals (in this article, these studies are referred to as acute studies). FormPro's database allows users to search by additional criteria to narrow results and to conduct specific searches for longitudinal studies, resources on life expectancy, resources that discuss the need for attendant care, and resources on employment after injury.

FormPro can also create questionnaires and checklists specifically for evidence-based life care planning. A Patient Care Needs Questionnaire can be created using specific criteria, including a patient's age, gender, and injury type. The questionnaire lists common medical services, surgical and procedural treatments, and diagnostic tests associated with a specific medical condition, as well as addressing a variety of other concerns applicable to the needs of a permanently impaired individual. The questionnaire has several sections that allow a provider or consultant to rate a patient's capacity for activities of daily living and their need for functional assistance.

A comprehensive list of complications of the specified injury appears near the end of the form, and the provider or consultant has the opportunity to rate each of them as potential, probable, or already present. A rating greater than 10% for any of the care needs, tests, complications, and so forth is the threshold level for inclusion on the form. A 10% threshold was believed to be adequate for inclusion for most circumstances, but additional comments are allowed, as noted in the forms. The FormPro checklist evolved from a desire to be thorough but also to eliminate undue influence by the life care planner.

The FormPro questionnaire and checklist system are flexible, allowing the user to add specific services warranted by a patient's needs and to omit any service deemed unnecessary. A key benefit of this flexibility is the ease with which a single questionnaire or checklist can be created to address more than 1 injury. If a patient has both a mild brain injury and complete paraplegia, for example, the user does not have to create a separate form for each condition. Instead of recording the opinions of physicians, consultants, and other care providers with the aid of documents created ad hoc, FormPro offers a standardized, repeatable, and comprehensive way of recording opinions for every case.

Determining Relevancy of Literature

Not all literature is of equal quality, and it is important to determine if an article is relevant to the case in question. In developing a life care plan, it is important to avoid animal studies, acute studies, and case studies. Animal studies are generally conducted as an initial step in experimental drug/procedure studies or to understand a process not yet understood in humans. The rational for conducting animal research is that it is safer or more ethical to test on animals before moving to humans; however, any information gleaned from animal studies would have to be confirmed by human studies to be empirically accepted as relevant in a human population. Although animal studies can be an important first step in research, they are not sufficient to make recommendations in a life care plan.

Acute studies often deal with short-term complications that resolve with time and treatment, or issues that are not present in an individual who is at maximum medical improvement. For example, many acute studies on traumatic brain injury focus on life-saving techniques, surgeries, therapies, and medications that are not relevant once 2 years has elapsed since the date of the person's brain injury. Although a certain therapy may prove beneficial during the acute stage, it may not be useful or provide any benefit once the acute stage of injury has passed. Case studies are generally useful only for rare disorders or injuries. For example, few if any large studies have been conducted on the long-term care needs of individuals with hemipelvectomy. Because the injury that requires a hemipelvectomy is itself rare, as is survival after the injury, a large population is not available to study for long-term care needs. Thus, in instances such as this, a case study may be able to provide the physician with some guidance where they would otherwise have little or none.

The ideal research investigation to support long-term care needs is a study with a large sample of individuals with the same injury at maximum medical improvement. Superior research chooses the appropriate design for the type of research being conducted. A sample that is as similar as possible to the individual being assessed is ideal, and matching demographic variables such as race, income level, and educational level make for an even more accurate fit. Literature reviews and meta-analyses are also good for synthesizing and assessing literature quality and applicability. Guidelines are statements to guide clinicians in decision making for a specific diagnosis or injury.[7] Guidelines usually include a review of the literature as well.

Greenhalgh[8] discusses the hierarchy of evidence when reviewing literature. At the top of the hierarchy and carrying the most weight are systematic reviews and meta-analyses. After systematic reviews are randomized controlled trials, cohort studies, case-control studies, and cross-sectional surveys. At the bottom of the hierarchy and carrying the least weight are case reports. However, not all studies lend themselves to a randomized controlled trial design, and not all randomized controlled studies are designed well. Some may have serious methodological flaws, limiting their applicability to a patient's specific condition.

THE PHYSIATRIST AS A CONSULTANT

Rehabilitation physicians are uniquely qualified to provide expert opinion for a life care plan by nature of their medical specialty. Through training, experience, and ongoing education, a physiatrist often provides lifelong care to individuals who have sustained an injury or illness that has resulted in a permanent impairment(s) and subsequent disabilities.[9] Once a physiatrist enters into a patient-physician relationship, they should be informally computing both the short-term and long-term care needs of the patient. In addition, physiatric care of a patient often overlaps and interfaces with care from multiple other health care providers, such as other physicians, allied health care providers, and complementary/alternative care practitioners. Accordingly, physiatric understanding of the holistic needs of a medically compromised patient arguably exceeds that of any other health care professional. Given their experience and qualifications, physiatrists are often sought by and develop professional relationships with life care planners, or in some cases even become life care planners. Incorporating skillful and knowledgeable physiatric expert opinion in a life care plan is a first step in ensuring that the plan is comprehensive and has appropriate medical foundation. For this article, it is assumed that the physiatrist is acting as a consultant to a life care planner, although the principles set forth here certainly are also applicable to physiatrist life care planners.

By acting as a consultant to a life care planner, the rehabilitation physician is providing expert opinion. Acting in such a capacity, the physiatrist typically falls into 1 of 4 categories. First, the physiatrist can be hired by a company or third party as an employee or more commonly as an independent contractor. The physiatrist in the later role characteristically is asked to perform an independent medical examination (IME) and then provide expert opinion based on that evaluation. Usually, such an arrangement occurs when the physiatrist has been hired on behalf of the defense. Second, the physiatrist may be hired by the plaintiff or injured party's representatives to provide expert opinion on their client's rehabilitation and therapy needs. Third, as a treating physician, the physiatrist may be asked to provide expert opinion on the current and future abilities and care needs of their patient. Fourth, and less frequent, the physiatrist may occasionally be hired by the court or by both parties involved in a medicolegal dispute to provide expert opinion commensurate with their expertise. In providing recommendations to a life care planner, it is assumed that the physiatrist has expertise in the area of dispute and provides opinions and conclusions without bias or prejudice. For this discussion, all but the treating physiatrist is referred to as the hired expert or simply as the expert, whereas the treating physiatrist is referred to as the treater.

As a treating physician, it is assumed the physiatrist has some level of expertise in the areas being addressed regarding their patient. As a consequence, the credential standards for the treating physician are not as rigorous as they are for the hired expert, who has not developed a treating relationship with the patient, client, or evaluee, but has been hired instead primarily for their ability and expertise in resolving a forensic matter. At a minimum, the hired expert should be in active medical practice, in which at least 50% of their time is spent in clinical practice, addressing the ongoing care needs of patients. The expert should be board certified and in good standing, with an unrestricted license. The expert also must have some level of clinical experience with the forensic matter on which they have been asked to provide opinions. A more detailed discussion of this topic is in Appendix 1 on proposed model code of conduct.

Ideally, the recommendations provided by either the treating physician or the hired expert are supported by the medical literature. However, often there may be a paucity or lack of applicable literature regarding a specific recommendation or opinion. Further, there may be no literature on a topic because the problem may be rare or difficult to study or, alternatively, the answer to the problem is self-evident. For example, it is self-evident to a physiatrist that a teenaged ambulating below-knee amputee requires a replacement leg or that a stroke survivor benefits from a shower chair and grab bars, thus no literature is needed to support these conclusions. If the opinions of the physiatrist related to a particular question deviate from accepted practice or findings in the literature, such opinions should be supported with rational foundation, so that anyone else considering the same question would come to the same conclusion more likely than not. That is, if the conclusions of the treater or expert differ from the literature or accepted practice, the expert should be prepared to explain the methodology on which they have relied to develop their conclusions. In the absence of good scientific data to support a particular conclusion or opinion, appropriate scientific methodology can be used instead. The physiatrist must have a basic understanding of the scientific method to formulate such conclusions.

Ethical Duties of the Physiatrist

One of the greatest pitfalls that the physiatrist may encounter when making recommendations for a life care plan is not recognizing leading questions or directly answering them. An example of a leading question is, "Wouldn't it be beneficial for Mr X to have a handicap-accessible van with adaptive equipment?" Certain assumptions need to be met for this to not be a leading question. For instance, is Mr X capable of driving, is Mr X incapable of performing a car transfer, and are attendants always available who can assist Mr X in his car transfers? Arguably, anyone who is a paraplegic would benefit from a handicap-accessible van, and why would one not outfit it with adaptive equipment, even if the paraplegic person cannot drive, because this person may have friends or peers who will use such equipment? However, not all paraplegics use handicap-accessible vans or require them. When confronted with such a question, the physiatrist should ask themselves whether such a vehicle is more likely than not medically necessary. Avoiding blanket approvals of such leading questions only strengthens the position of the treater or expert. Using a checklist, like those available through FormPro, eliminates the potential for bias or undue influence of the life care planner on the consulting physiatry expert. In addition, for those physiatrists who also prepare life care plans, using the FormPro checklist underscores the methodology that physiatrists use when thinking about their patient's or client's long-term care needs and when formulating a treatment plan. FormPro puts on paper the thought process that good physiatrists use when they interview and examine a particular patient.

When providing opinions and conclusions, the physiatrist obviously relies on their skill, knowledge, training, education, and clinical experience. However, what matters most in the medicolegal world is scientific data to support these conclusions. Thus, solely keeping current on the literature is insufficient. The expert and treater must have a thorough understanding of the literature as it applies to the forensic matter at hand, and they should understand the scientific merits of each applicable study and the particular strengths and weakness of the investigators' conclusions.

EVIDENCED-BASED OPINION AND THE DAUBERT DECISION

The importance of an evidence-based opinion in life care plans was underscored by the Daubert decision, Daubert v Merrell Dow Pharmaceuticals, 509 US 579, 589 (1993).[10] Physiatrists who provide expert opinion on life care plans that are to be presented in a legal context must adhere to the Daubert standard. Daubert states:

A witness who is qualified as an expert by knowledge, skill, experience, training, or education may testify in the form of an opinion or otherwise if:
a. The expert's scientific, technical, or other specialized knowledge helps the trier of fact to understand the evidence or to determine a fact in issue;
b. The testimony is based on sufficient facts or data;
c. The testimony is the product of reliable principles and methods; and,
d. The expert has reliably applied the principles and methods to the facts of the case.

The valuable role that a physiatrist can play when producing an accurate life care plan and the importance of using appropriate literature to further support the physiatrist's opinions and conclusions whenever possible have been summarized. A thoughtful, well-trained, experienced physiatrist who draws support from relevant literature exceeds the Daubert standard. In medicine, relative to the range of potential problems a patient may have, there is a paucity of research available. Thus, applying the Daubert standard to all recommendations given to a life care planner who is attempting to develop an accurate plan is not always possible. Further, for self-evident needs, the Daubert standard does not need to be met (an example is hand controls for a paraplegic driver).

SUMMARY

When providing opinions and conclusions for a life care plan, the physiatrist has entered the world of medicolegal or forensic medicine. If such opinions are requested by the defendant or insurer, the physiatrist may evaluate the client by performing an IME. As a treater, the knowledge required to provide expert opinion may already be at hand or derived from the doctor's chart notes. As a plaintiff nontreater expert, an examination similar to an IME also needs to be performed. Regardless of which side has solicited the expert opinion, the physiatrist has certain ethical obligations, which are reviewed in detail in Appendix 1. The duties of a physiatrist working in such a medicolegal capacity should not be taken lightly. The respectful sacred trust that develops in a patient-physician relationship should be extended into the medicolegal arena.

REFERENCES

1. Law M, MacDermid J, editors. Evidence-based rehabilitation: a guide to practice. 2nd edition. Thorofare (NJ): Slack; 2008.
2. CINAHL Plus with Full Text. EBSCO Publishing. Available at: http://www.ebscohost.com/academic/cinahl-plus-with-full-text/.

3. American Psychological Association. APA PsycNET. Available at: http://www.apa. org/pubs/databases/psycnet/index.aspx.

4. National Center for Biotechnology Information. US National Library of Medicine. National Institutes of Health. PubMed. Available at: http://www.ncbi.nlm.nih.gov/ pubmed.

5. Elsevier. Available at: http://www.elsevier.com/.

6. Brightsun Technologies. FormPro. Available at: http://www.brightsuntech.com/ FormPro.aspx.

7. Straus SE, Richardson WS, Glasziou P, et al. Evidence-based medicine: how to practice and teach EBM. 3rd edition. Philadelphia: Elsevier; 2005.

8. Greenhalgh T. How to read a paper. Getting your bearings (deciding what the paper is about). BMJ 1997;315(7102):243–6.

9. Weed RO, Berens DE. Life care planning and case management handbook. 3rd edition. Boca Raton (FL): CRC Press; 2010.

10. Daubert v Merrell Dow Pharmaceuticals (92-102), 509 US 579. 1993.

APPENDIX 1: PROPOSED MODEL CODE OF CONDUCT
Introduction

This proposed model code of conduct, hereafter referred to as the Code, is a first step in providing ethical guidelines for physiatrists performing IMEs, providing expert opinion for life care plans, or expressing opinions and conclusions in medicolegal matters.

Physicians who provide expert opinion on a medicolegal matter typically fall into 1 of 3 categories: an expert hired by the defense, an expert hired by the plaintiff, or a treating physician (treater). At times, the treating physician also is designated as an expert. For this discussion, the treater is also referred to as expert.

In the ideal situation, both litigating parties would agree on and be equally financially responsible for a single medical evaluator. In this scenario, the physician has a greater potential to be truly independent. Despite the rarity of such circumstances, the evaluator in this case would be held to the same ethical standards as any other physician performing medicolegal work. Regardless of the source of referral, the ethical duties of the physician performing medicolegal work are equivalent. Opinions and conclusions should be provided in an unbiased and respectful manner, consistently based on objective findings and, when possible, supported by medical literature.

Because of the relationship with their own contracted employers, an independent medical examiner ethically is no different from an insurance or company physician. Both types of physicians have financial contractual obligations with an insurer, the insurer's representative, or a business. Similarly, the treating physician may have potential conflicts between their perceived fiduciary duty to the patient and duty toward the court. The physiatrist performing medicolegal services has a duty to recognize the pressures, such as financial incentives, religious beliefs, cultural habits, political leanings, and so forth, that can lead to bias. Every attempt needs to be made to avoid such prejudices. A treating physician cannot act as an expert for either party without the express consent of their patient, even if their relationship has lapsed.

In the Code, the terms *must* and *should* are used in the following ways:

- *Must* denotes an overriding duty or principle.
- *Should* is used to provide an explanation on how overriding duty is met or when the duty or principle does not apply in all situations or circumstances, or when factors outside the control of the evaluator affect compliance with the Code.

When the term expertist is used in the Code, it refers to the medicolegal evaluator acting in the capacity of an expert witness. The Code must not be interpreted as a declaration of evaluator or evaluee rights, nor should it be construed as legal advice. The Code is a proposed guide for medicolegal evaluators to avoid ethical and legal dilemmas when conducting evaluations or expressing opinions and conclusions. The more expansive the Code, the greater the difficulty in meeting all of the proposed guidelines. Not all guidelines may be applicable in all situations. The goal of this model is to set forth comprehensive guidelines that avoid omissions. Many of the responsibilities and duties outlined in this proposal are not necessarily consistently applicable. In addition, certain diagnoses cannot always be objectified, such as many pain syndromes, particularly headaches. However, the physiatrist performing medicolegal work should be able to recognize their standing within each of the 6 areas of responsibility.

The Code encompasses 6 areas of responsibility:

A. Fundamental responsibilities
B. Responsibilities to evaluee (client/patient)
C. Responsibilities to society and the court
D. Responsibilities to the referring party
E. Responsibilities to other experts and treating professionals
F. Responsibilities to oneself

Fundamental responsibilities

1. Must recognize the overarching duty of experts to the court, statutory and regulatory law, and the common law decisions of the courts.
2. Must demonstrate rigor and sound methodology.
3. Must understand that the evaluator's role must focus on the following:
   a. Search for and identification of facts
   b. Validation of the evaluee's complaint(s)
   c. Performance of a quality clinical evaluation
   d. Unbiased interpretation of relevant investigations and data
   e. Formulation of a considered opinion.
4. Must take reasonable steps to secure access to evidence and documentation, review all relevant evidence and documentation, and identify missing data and their importance.
5. Must objectively, accurately, and impartially document, corroborate, and use scientific and clinical methodology(ies) to critically review the data, facts, and evaluee's health claim, injury/disease, impairment, activity limitation, social participation restriction, and contextual factors, among others.
6. Must show objectivity by:
   a. Documenting relevant facts
   b. Corroborating statements
   c. Comparing the evaluee's reported loss with the available evidence (eg, examination for discovery, observations made on direct examination, laboratory findings, diagnostic tests, other evaluations, surveillance).
7. Must perform a competent comprehensive quality history taking that includes relevant, precise and detailed information as reported spontaneously by the evaluee and in response to direct inquiry. Must supplement and contrast this history with existing documented evidence, as necessary pursuant to the mandate.
8. Must perform a complete and detailed physical evaluation, including precise descriptions and measurements, when indicated.

9. Must provide fair, objective, and nonpartisan data and opinion. Must not show complacency, advocacy for the claimant or referring party, overt skepticism, or distrust.
10. Must be honest and trustworthy in all verbal and written statements throughout the medicolegal evaluation and expert testimony process.
11. Must take reasonable steps to verify the accuracy of signed reports, forms, and documents. Must corroborate the information provided by the evaluee and provide comment if relevant information has been excluded or discounted.
12. Must not allow views about any individual's age, color, culture, disability, ethnic or national origin, gender, lifestyle, marital or parental status, race, religion or beliefs, sex, sexual orientation, or social or economic status to prejudice the evidence.
13. Must use language and terminology readily understood by those requesting the expert opinion. Abbreviations, medical, and other technical terminology should be defined or explained.
14. Must use plain, logical, and fallacy-free fact-supported arguments.
15. Must keep current in area of practice and adhere to the laws, civil rules of procedures, and regulatory policies that affect third-party assessments or expert witnessing.

Responsibilities to the evaluee

General responsibilities
1. Must introduce oneself to the evaluee and explain the nature, purpose, and process of the evaluation, and provide the identities of the referring party and the recipient of the evaluation report.
2. Must take reasonable steps to address any perceived inconsistencies in the documentation with the evaluee. Reviewing documentation before the evaluation is deemed as best practice.
3. Must act with integrity, civility, and professionalism and must show respect for the evaluee's dignity and autonomy. This responsibility includes the evaluee's right to privacy during dressing/undressing and on examination.
4. Must endeavor to provide a healthy and safe environment for the evaluee, office personnel, and oneself. Must not engage in hostile behavior, physical or verbal abuse, violence, or harassment of any kind. The evaluation must be terminated if any such behavior by any of the parties involved occurs.
5. Must communicate effectively and clearly about all elements related to the medicolegal evaluation and report process. Must warn the evaluee of any testing that may elicit pain or discomfort and document it when it occurs. Must inform the evaluee that they have the prerogative to refuse any aspect of the examination, particularly if they believe a portion of the examination may be injurious.
6. Must bring to the evaluee's attention any serious medical health condition not previously diagnosed and advise the evaluee to seek appropriate medical attention. In the case of a medical emergency, reasonable steps must be taken to inform the treating physician. This information should be included in the report to the requesting party.
7. Must avoid any comments irrelevant to the mandate.
8. Must prepare an addendum report to correct/amend any material factual or legal errors.
9. Must provide reasonable accommodation for persons with a disability, language, or communication barrier. Interpretation services should preferably be provided by a professional having no relationship with the evaluee.

Initiating an evaluee-evaluator relationship
1. Must explain the nature and extent of the evaluator's responsibility to the referring source or the court. Must underscore the absence of a treating relationship.
2. Must warn the evaluee that any information provided can be included in the report to the referring party.

Communication and consent
1. Should obtain oral and written informed consent to perform the evaluation and release the report(s) or discuss findings with the referring party. Examples of written consent/agreements can be found in Appendix 2.
2. Must explain that the report will be submitted to the requesting party and that, unless duly specified, a copy of the report can be obtained only from the party the report belongs to unless this duty to the referring party is waived.
3. Must obtain specific authorization from the evaluee to take pictures or make an audio or video recording of the evaluation.
4. Must explain to the evaluee that withdrawing or not providing consent can negatively affect the evaluee's benefits status or compensatory awards.

Privacy and confidentiality
1. Must explain to the evaluee that any personal health information can and may be disclosed to the requesting party and otherwise kept confidential unless a legal requirement permits or requires disclosing any such information to another party.
2. Must take all reasonable steps to maintain integrity and security of all health records.

Responsibilities to society and the court

1. Must prepare a report, when asked, compliant with the relevant rules of the court or adjudicative body (ie, an expert witness disclosure).
2. Must accurately describe the evaluator's education, training, skills, experience, qualifications, positions, and responsibilities.
3. Must make clear the scope of the evaluator's knowledge or competence. Should make clear during expert testimony when a particular question or issue falls outside the scope of practice or expertise.
4. Must understand and follow the rule of evidence regarding the admissibility of scientific expert testimony. Should be familiar with the Daubert standard.
5. Must state that opinions are provisional or qualified in situations in which data are missing or are materially insufficient and, therefore, findings are subject to change.
6. If asked, must provide a rationale and explanation for all opinions and conclusions and state supporting facts or assumptions, including relevant clinical or scientific references.
7. Must be prepared to provide literature, when such literature is known and available, to support the opinions and conclusions of the expert, and if contrary literature is obtainable, be prepared to explain why such literature is not applicable to the circumstances at hand.
8. Must render such additional assistance as the court or adjudicative body may reasonably require when determining a matter in issue. The expert's duty to the court or adjudicative body overrides the obligation to the retaining party.
9. Must provide an opinion based on supporting facts or assumptions. Should summarize the range of opinion and, if asked, explain how one's view was arrived at

and be prepared to reject alternative views by providing relevant facts, clinical, or scientific references. Must consider all material facts that do not support the concluded opinion.

10. Must correctly apply the civil standard of proof to both factual and opinion evidence. This statement means there is more than 50% probability or chance (ie, is more likely than not) that the accident or adverse event caused the injuries or loss complained of.

11. Must understand that the application of the material contribution principle can be applied in only limited circumstances. The most common application is in occupational diseases. The material contribution test is generally applied to a claim in which 2 or more potential causative factors are responsible for a condition. Three important distinguishing factors are present in all cases in which the material contribution causation test should be applied:
   a. The agent or activity responsible for causing the disease or condition is the same in each of several periods of exposure;
   b. The mechanism by which that agent or activity is applied to the claimant is the same or nearly the same;
   c. Medical science cannot prove which period of exposure caused the injury.

12. Must apportion damages, when possible, if presented with a claim for which there is preexisting or intervening condition(s) or claim(s). Should be prepared to explain methodology in deriving such apportionment.

13. Must use the following terms when addressing causation: probable (more than 50%), not probable or possible (less than 50%), certain (100%), and impossible (0%). Terms such as plausible, likely, and conceivable should be avoided.

14. Must understand the distinction in the medicolegal use of the terms injury, symptoms, impairments, effects/limitations, and consequences/sequelae, which are defined as follows:
   Injury: the physical/psychological trauma suffered
   Symptoms: the physical/psychological manifestations of the injury
   Impairment: the loss or loss of use of a body part, structure, or organ
   Effects/limitations: the physical/psychological limitations experienced by the claimant as a result of the injury/symptoms
   Consequences/sequelae: the restrictions on the activities of daily living, now and for the future, that result from the injury/symptoms/effects.

15. Must understand the difference between the words exacerbation, acceleration, and aggravation in the medicolegal context. Exacerbation refers to a time-limited increase in symptoms of a preexisting condition after an event. An exacerbation is often also referred to as a temporary aggravation. Acceleration applies to a condition in which the level of symptoms of a preexisting condition has been brought forward in time. Aggravation refers to a new permanent injury or additional loss, when there was already a preexisting condition.

16. Should be prepared to offer evidence addressing not only what the consequences of an injury on the evaluee's capabilities are, and will be, but also what would have occurred in the evaluee's life in the absence of the injury sustained. Must describe the possibility of complications (preferably using percentages) after an injury to assist the estimation of future damages. Must also apply the reasonable foreseeability principle to current and probable future damages.

17. Must apply the legal test of real and substantial probable risk for considering future care (medical cost projections or life care plans). The future care need must also be shown to be reasonably necessary on the medical evidence. This statement means that an objective analysis of each individual item must be

conducted to determine whether the item is medically justified, reasonably necessary, and not merely beneficial.

18. Must apply the proper standard of proof for future pecuniary costs, which is a real and substantial risk.
19. Must use a clear methodology when addressing a causal relationship. This methodology should include the following:
    a. A specialized inquiry to establish the evaluee's preexisting health, functioning, and disablement state and validate it with the available evidence. The presence of a condition that meets the eggshell client theory should be identified (ie, identify those evaluees who are mentally or physically fragile for whom injuries may cause disproportionate symptoms and impairment).
    b. Identify the presence of coexisting and intervening factors or events contributing to the evaluee's current health, functioning, and disablement.
    c. Take into consideration the natural history of the disease or injury, the known complications, and associated disablement.
    d. Validate the reality, nature, and severity of the trauma or disease.
    e. Address the mechanism of injury and disablement.
    f. Address any delay of onset of the symptoms, disease, and disablement.
    g. Address the continuity and progression of the complaints.
    h. Evaluate congruency between the site of injury, impairment, and disablement.
20. Must describe the nature, duration, and seriousness of the specific hazard(s) or risk(s) that justify a medically required work absence or restriction.
21. Must immediately report to the referring party or the court any issues of duress when the evaluator is subjected to or threatened with violence, legal action, recrimination, reprisal, constraints, or other action by another party.
22. Must be able to identify the set of criteria used to render a specific diagnosis.
23. Must be familiar with, if known, the potential error rate of the methods or tests relied on to formulate an opinion.
24. Must address situations in which exaggeration, deception, simulation, fabrication, or malingering is suspected.
25. Must address issues of noncompliance with treatment recommendations.
26. Should indicate when a treatment regime is outside the generally accepted norms or is potentially harmful.

Responsibilities to the referring party

1. Must declare any real, potential, or perceived direct or indirect conflict of interest with the evaluee and request direction from the referring party.
2. Must adopt clear conflict-of-interest or disclosure policies regarding physicians and insurance companies or law firms.
3. Must disclose any previous treating relationship with the evaluee. Information obtained in the course of the treating relationship should not be used in third-party assessment without the patient's consent.
4. Must provide any report, form, document, signature, or evidence that the evaluator has agreed to produce, unless the contractual agreement with the referring party has been terminated or the evaluator has been instructed by the referring party to do otherwise.
5. Must ensure that the mandate and questions are clear and seek clarification if the instructions are unclear, inadequate, or conflicting. In the case of unclear instructions, an expert opinion should not be provided.
6. Must ensure that all questions posed by the requesting party have been addressed.

7. Must deal only with matters within the limits of one's professional expertise, direct experience, and competency and decline those outside the area of expertise or for which there is insufficient information. Curbside opinions from other physicians should not be incorporated into an expert's opinions or conclusions. If a particular area is not addressed, the reasons for this should be clearly stated.
8. The expert or treater should be aware of the standards of care and nature of practice at the time of the incident. Must understand that acceptance of a medicolegal mandate implies a willingness to act as an expert witness.
9. Must provide to the referring party reasonable and customary fees for the nature, duration, and complexity of the service rendered, in advance. Must not accept contingencies fees or enter into fee-splitting arrangements. Retainer fees are permissible. The evaluator should provide a reasonable explanation or breakdown that allows the referring party to understand the invoice.
10. Must explain any limitations when providing an opinion about an individual without the opportunity to consult or examine that individual.
11. Must identify relevant nonmedical issues but refrain from commenting on these if outside the field of expertise. Should recognize that health can be best assessed using a comprehensive biopsychosocial approach or model.
12. Must inform the referring party without delay if facts or opinions have materially changed.
13. Must inform the requesting party of any unforeseen delay in providing an opinion or a report.

Responsibilities to other experts and treating professionals

1. Must avoid disparaging comments relative to other health care professionals' treatments, opinions, or reports and not engage in personal attacks when commenting on another expert's divergent opinions or views.
2. Must identify assessments or treatment interventions that do not meet standard of care or may be fraudulent.
3. Must provide detailed and balanced argumentation based on facts and scientific evidence to qualify another expert opinion.
4. Must uphold the Code for oneself and others.

Responsibilities to oneself

1. Must keep current and be clinically active in the chosen field of expertise and specialized knowledge.
2. Must maintain competence and proficiency in the medicolegal field by participating in continuing professional education and peer review.
3. Must advocate for the development and safeguard of the highest medicolegal standard of practice.
4. Must resist any influence or interference that could undermine the evaluator's professional integrity.
5. Must recognize that the evaluator's physical and emotional health and well-being can affect the medicolegal practice.

Summary

We hope that this proposed model for ethical behavior generates discussions and leads to the development and adoption of guidelines for physiatrists through an organizational body, such as the American Academy of Physical Medicine and Rehabilitation. We welcome any suggestions, assistance, or guidance toward meeting this goal or in improving this model. We expect this document to evolve over time as our role in the medicolegal field becomes better defined and the knowledge base of rehabilitation medicine expands.

APPENDIX 2: SAMPLE WRITTEN INFORMED CONSENT

PLAINTIFF MEDICAL AGREEMENT

I understand that _____, MD, has been asked by _____ to provide opinions and conclusions regarding various aspects of my medical condition, as it relates to his specialty, Physical Medicine and Rehabilitation. I understand that the opinions and conclusions of _____, MD, are his alone and may not necessarily reflect my personal views and thoughts regarding my condition.

I authorize and release _____, MD, to discuss information relating to my condition, for the purposes as outlined above.

_____
Date

_____
Signature Evaluee/Client/Patient

INDEPENDENT MEDICAL EXAMINATION AGREEMENT

I understand that I am undergoing an examination by a physician hired by the defendant/insurer. I understand that _____, MD will NOT serve as my primary or consulting physician. I understand that NO patient–physician relationship will be established and I waive any rights normally associated with such a relationship.

I understand that the report of _____, MD will be based on my history and physical examination, past medical history, and the records available for the doctor's review. I understand that _____'s opinions and conclusions are being solicited by the defendant/insurer.

I authorize and release _____, MD, to discuss information concerning the results of the medical examination, for the purposes as outlined above.

_____
Date

_____
Signature Evaluee/Client/Patient

Index

Note: Page numbers of article titles are in **boldface** type.

Phys Med Rehabil Clin N Am 24 (2013) 567–572
http://dx.doi.org/10.1016/S1047-9651(13)00043-0
1047-9651/13/$ – see front matter © 2013 Elsevier Inc. All rights reserved.

pmr.theclinics.com

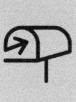

Printed and bound by CPI Group (UK) Ltd, Croydon, CR0 4YY

03/10/2024

01040465-0018